Success with your insulin pump

A Successful Diabetes Handbook

Jill Rodgers

Published by SD Publications, Successful Diabetes, PO Box 819, Northampton NN4 4AG

ISBN 978-1-4477-3548-9

This book contains practical advice about managing diabetes. Every effort has been made to ensure that the information contained in this book is accurate, but it is not intended to replace individual medical advice. If you have diabetes, and you are in any doubt, please discuss with your health professionals whether the recommendations in this book will work for you and your diabetes.

Contents

Contents (continued)

About Us

Successful Diabetes is an independent company run by health professionals who are education specialists. They provide products and services to benefit those working or living with diabetes and other long term conditions.

They offer a wide range of products including books and ebooks, workshops and website resources such as recipes and practical tips on all aspects of living and working with diabetes.

The author of this book is Jill Rodgers, one of the Directors of Successful Diabetes. Jill is a former diabetes specialist nurse who has several years experience of starting many people with diabetes on pump therapy, and has also helped diabetes teams set up pump services.

Jill also wrote the first-ever UK insulin pump book 'Using insulin pumps – a practical guide for nurses and other health professionals', published by John Wiley and Sons Ltd in 2008.

Acknowledgements

I would like to thank the many insulin pump users who have influenced the content of this book, including those whom I have personally helped with using insulin pumps, and those whom I've got to know through my work in diabetes. All have willingly shared both their positive and negative experiences and also their feelings, and many of the quotes in this book have been taken from information they have willingly shared with me to enable others to understand the reality of pump therapy better. Thank you.

Introduction

Insulin pump therapy is becoming an increasingly popular option in the treatment of Type 1 diabetes and, in a more limited way, Type 2 diabetes. However, it does not suit everyone, and nor will every person with diabetes want to use a pump if it is offered to them. It can be difficult to make a decision about whether an insulin pump is something you would like to use when you have very limited knowledge about them. This book is written with adults with diabetes in mind, but many of the ideas can also be used by parents and children.

Changing from using insulin injections to pump therapy is definitely a trip outside your comfort zone, and it may cause you anxiety or worries, or make you feel like a beginner again. This book will provide you with basic information to refer back to about all aspects of pump therapy, particularly how you might manage your diabetes differently than you did before you had a pump. As you get more used to your pump, this book will also help you experiment with your insulin doses using a pump, and gain confidence in dealing with potentially challenging situations.

If you are thinking of getting a pump, just starting out with using one, or have been using pump therapy for some time, there will be something in this book for you. Chapters one and two explain what pump therapy is and provide help and advice for those of you who have not yet got an insulin pump, including useful information on where to go for help and support if you are finding it difficult to obtain a pump. You can also read about how to prepare for the day you start using a pump for the first time.

Chapters three and four are essential reading if you are just starting to use a pump, and are designed to be read in conjunction with each other. They will take you step by step through how to set your initial insulin pump infusion rates, both basal rates and bolus doses, and also help you think about the practical and psychological aspects of using a pump that you will need to think about during the early days.

Chapters five and six deal specifically with how to manage high and low blood glucose levels and how to adjust your insulin doses proactively to help you get the best out of your pump. Some of this information can be useful as you start out with a pump, or you can revisit it at times when you feel things aren't working as well as they should be.

Chapter seven discusses different aspects of living with your pump, and chapter eight provides some frequently asked questions about pump therapy that are not answered elsewhere in the book.

Overall, this book is your practical companion for information, ideas and confidence, wherever you are on your insulin pump journey. Happy reading and good luck!

Chapter 1: Understanding pump therapy

What is insulin pump therapy?

Insulin pump therapy, officially called continuous subcutaneous insulin infusion (CSII) therapy, is simply a method of giving insulin continuously rather than as a series of injections at different times of the day. Most pumps consist of the pump itself which holds a reservoir of insulin, a length of tubing, and a small device (a cannula) attached to the length of tubing which is inserted into your body to allow the insulin in. This type of pump may be programmed by pressing buttons on the pump itself or by using a wireless electronic programming device. There are also 'patch pumps', where the insulin is in a reservoir at the cannula site, with no tubing and a wireless electronic programming device.

The rationale behind using an insulin pump is that it delivers insulin in a far more physiological way, which means that it can more closely copy the way that you would produce insulin from your own pancreas. Therefore, you programme a small amount of insulin to be delivered in tiny quantities through each hour of the day, and you can vary the amount at different times of the day depending on your needs. You can give extra doses of insulin at any time, most commonly to match any carbohydrate-containing food you are eating, but also if you are unwell or have other reasons for your blood glucose level being higher than normal. This means that you can control your blood glucose more tightly, rather than waiting for the next injection to correct any high readings. Likewise, you can reduce the dose at any point if you need less insulin, such as when you increase your activity levels for a short or longer time.

The pros and cons of insulin pumps

Many people, whether they live or work with diabetes, have strong and often diverse opinions about whether using an insulin pump is a positive step, and this variety of opinion can make it hard to make an objective decision. For those living with diabetes, some will have found that their pump has revolutionised their life in a very positive way; for others, it may not have been such a success story. Some health professionals will recommend insulin pump therapy as a positive treatment choice, and some may feel it should only be used when nothing else has worked. Here you'll find information about the pros and cons, including real-life examples, to help you with your decision.

The positive side: Why insulin pumps are great

Enthusiasts of insulin pumps will give you lots of reasons why they think pumps are great, all of them valid. Take a look and see what you think of the reasons they might share with you about the positive aspects of insulin pump therapy.

No more injections

This is one of the most popular attractions of using an insulin pump! Rapid acting insulin is delivered continuously through a small needle or cannula, and the rate can be varied to meet your needs. So whilst needles are still involved, once you have inserted the needle or cannula, unless there are any problems with the site (for example redness or blockage), you only need to replace it every two or three days.

Your insulin pump can be programmed to suit you, and you can give extra insulin at any point by pressing the buttons on your pump. However, using an insulin pump is not an absolute guarantee that you will never need another injection. If you are unwell and your blood glucose levels reach high levels and do not seem to be responding to the insulin you are giving, you would need to give insulin using an insulin pen or syringe. Also, if the pump appeared to be malfunctioning in any way, you may need to go back to injections temporarily whilst it is sorted out. But both of these scenarios are likely to be rare and also short-term, so that once they have been resolved, you would be able to resume using your insulin pump.

It feels like freedom! Not having to inject at night time is strangely liberating!

Insulin works more predictably

Almost all the configurations of how you can take insulin by injection include some sort of longer-acting insulin. There are a number of newer versions of these, called long-acting analogues, which are much more sophisticated and predictable than their predecessors, but you will still get some unpredictable variation in how they work over a 24 hour period. An insulin pump only gives rapid acting insulin, so the variability of insulin release that comes from longer-acting types of insulin is removed.

I really wanted a pump because although I've always had good control, the price has been frequent hypos

Feeling more successful and confident

An insulin pump can help you to gain control over your diabetes, rather than it controlling you. You might be able to do activities you previously avoided because they used to give you a hypo. You might be able to do your job better, or do different social activities, feeling confident that you can fine tune your insulin dose adjustments to keep your blood glucose level balanced.

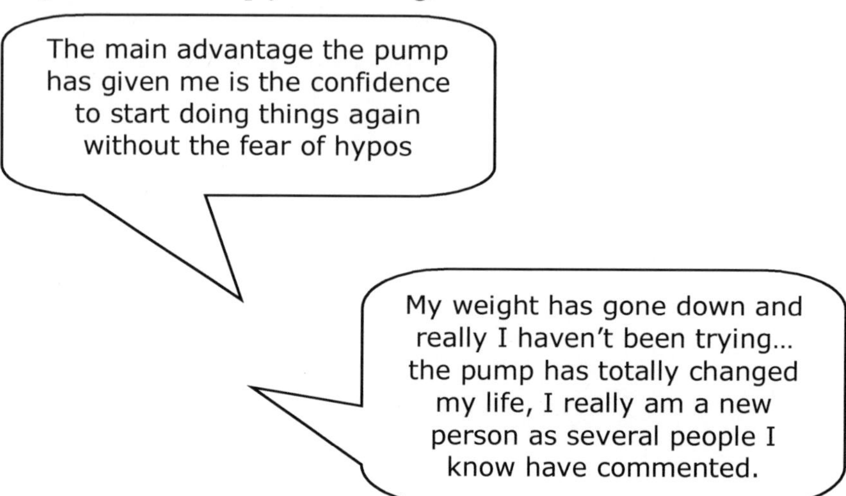

If you find yourself in a situation where your blood glucose is too high or too low, you can immediately alter your insulin dose and feel confident that it will work. Small numbers of people still find it difficult to manage and control their diabetes with an insulin pump, but most feel as though they 'get their lives back'.

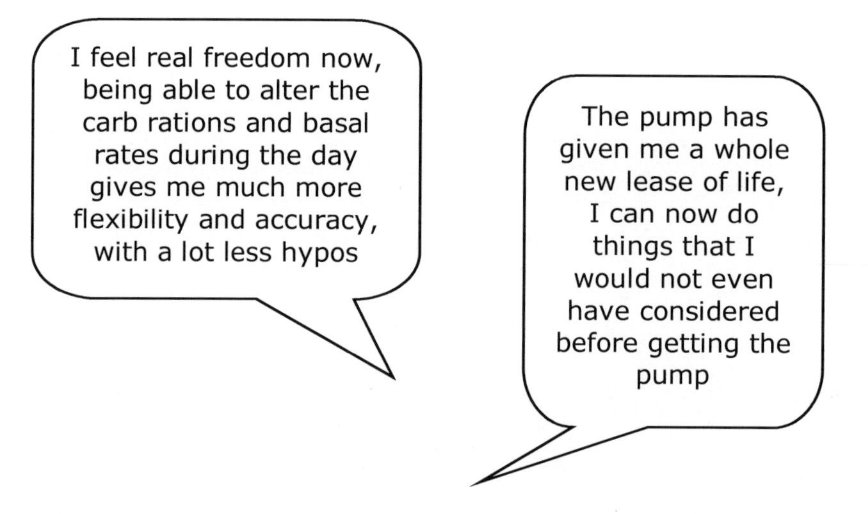

Improved HbA1c levels

The National Institute of Health and Clinical Excellence (NICE) recommendations on the level of HbA1c at which a pump should be considered (see page 23) support the concept that it is a way of reducing your HbA1c level. Whilst this does not work for everyone, it does for the majority, and some people experience quite dramatic reductions. This is partly because the day to day fluctuations in blood glucose readings tends to reduce, and as a result the average readings improve. Alongside the personal and lifestyle positive aspects of pump therapy, this medical effect is an important aspect.

I went back to the clinic and for once I was looking forward to it - and my HbA1c had dropped in two months from 9.9% to 7.9%! My consultant and nurse were thrilled!

Less planning ahead

If you have injections, it can be difficult to change your plans on the spur of the moment, especially your food or level of activity. With a pump, although you sometimes need to plan ahead, most of the time you can suddenly change your plans and change your insulin dose to match. As a result, eating and drinking and physical activity are all made easier – see the relevant sections below for more information.

Easier to manage physical activity

For physical activity, such as attending an exercise class or playing football, your insulin dose can be reduced a relatively short time beforehand, or you can remove the pump for an hour. If you need to, you can also set or continue a reduced insulin dose for a period after you have finished your activity. The amount you reduce your dose, and the length of time you set the reduced dose for, are both chosen by you so that you can match the changes to your personal situation.

For less strenuous activity which can still make a difference to your blood glucose level, such as housework, shopping or light gardening, you can make small adjustments to your insulin at any point to make sure that your blood glucose level doesn't drop too low. In general, being able to reduce your insulin in this way means that you don't need to eat as many snacks to avoid hypoglycaemia (hypo). With competitive sports or strenuous sports, both an insulin reduction and additional carbohydrates are likely to be needed, and more careful planning is required.

> Going to the gym is much easier – by reducing my basal rate temporarily I have for the first time been able to avoid post exercise hypos!

Eat what you like, when you like

You may have attended a structured education programme to help you with managing your diabetes, and for those with Type 1 diabetes, it will have included ways of eating flexibly and tailoring your insulin doses and injections to match. That approach offers a lot more options of how to successfully manage your diabetes, but insulin pumps can provide even more. For example:

- You never have to give yourself extra insulin in advance for a snack you might want in an hour or two's time – you simply press the buttons to give yourself the insulin you need at the time you need it
- You should rarely have to eat food to catch up with the insulin you have already injected
- All your insulin doses can be very quickly adjusted to match your food, including being able to give yourself a small amount of insulin with every course when you are eating out. If you are uncertain about the amount of insulin you need, it is easy to give a little less and then add more a couple of hours later if it hasn't quite controlled your blood glucose level enough.

The downside of using an insulin pump

Wearing the pump 24/7

Wearing a pump 24 hours a day is a big step to take, and it is common to experience feelings of not wanting to be attached to a machine 24 hours a day. It can feel as though your diabetes is made visible or feels more 'medical', rather than you being able to discretely give injections.

It may also affect your relationships, for example your partner might feel strongly negative towards you being attached to a machine. You could also be concerned about sleeping with a pump – for example, wondering if you will accidentally press buttons and give additional insulin, or if it will become disconnected during the night.

In reality, pumps can be easily concealed, and don't cause problems at night for the majority of people, but these concerns might be enough for some to make a choice not to wear a pump. If you are worried about any aspect of wearing the pump, share your concerns with your diabetes team and if possible with other pump users who can tell you about their experiences. If you are still not happy, a pump probably isn't for you.

> I had a number of concerns, not least that I would be permanently attached to a machine

Hard work

In the early days, it can feel as though your insulin pump is taking over your life. It definitely isn't something that you can leave to look after itself, and a lot of hard work is required to work out the insulin you need, test your blood glucose a lot, and work out how you can programme your pump to fit into the different situations in your life. Most pump users report that in time the work gets a lot easier as you become more confident about what to do and what results you will get. Although the initial work in the first couple of weeks does reduce in time, most say that it takes about six months to really get used to it and be able to make good decisions most of the time.

It can take a lot of perseverance to eventually see the different a pump can make. Once you have achieved what you want, there is still a reasonable amount of work to do on a daily basis, but it becomes more worthwhile as you can gain confidence in what you will achieve as a result.

It can change your life in so many ways but you do have to be committed and be prepared to work hard

I was told that the only downfall was the fact that I would have to test my blood more often than I was doing, but that's a small price to pay for better control

Insecurity

Even if injecting insulin isn't giving you the best blood glucose control, it is a familiar system that you know about, and it can feel quite uncomfortable to try a different system. You might be worried about losing the pump, or it becoming detached from you and you don't get enough insulin, or simply that you won't know what to do. It is a completely different system, which is why it needs so much attention at the beginning – some pump users report it was much easier than they thought it would be, whereas others say that they hadn't realised how different it would be. It can feel like learning about diabetes all over again, and can make you feel very insecure.

> Part of the reason why I resisted getting a pump was that I don't like changing stuff, and I had a sort of system going. Also, I sort of like being in control and didn't want to feel like a beginner

No days off

You might feel that using a pump will mean 'no days off' from diabetes. Whilst this is true for diabetes in general – you can't just give it away for a day! – when you use injection therapy, you can potentially have days when you give your diabetes very little thought. You may reach this stage once you're used to a pump too, but in general there is more thinking involved. Many pump users report that although they feel they are less able to forget about or ignore their diabetes at times, they feel that the benefits they gain (not just immediate but to their long term health) mean that it is a positive experience and much less stressful than managing diabetes with injections.

What if it doesn't work for me?

> I was informed that they would need to see if I was an acceptable candidate, and that if it didn't work I would be taken off it

Even though you may be committed to the pump and see that it has advantages, the actual experience of wearing it may make you realise it is not for you. This can be a difficult realisation, especially if you have been through a lot to obtain a pump, for example campaigning, having assessments or being on a waiting list. You may also feel pressured to make it work or you will have to have injections again.

It is important to remember that an insulin pump is simply one method of taking insulin – one of the tools that are part of the 'diabetes toolkit' – and it can be tried and given back if you feel that it is not working for you, whatever impression you have been given. Deciding to go back to insulin injections still leaves you with the option of considering using a pump again in the future.

Affecting your whole life?

You may be worried about how other parts of your life might be affected by using a pump, for example holidays, physical activity, social occasions and relationships. Most people's experiences are positive once they have grasped the general principles and how to manage situations differently using a pump instead of injections. The general principles of insulin pump therapy are the same as any other therapy, with the key questions being "what do I need to do to make my blood sugars rise, or make them fall, or keep them the same?" An insulin pump provides a better opportunity to more closely match your insulin to your life, but there is some work involved in finding out what works for you, particularly in the early days of using an insulin pump.

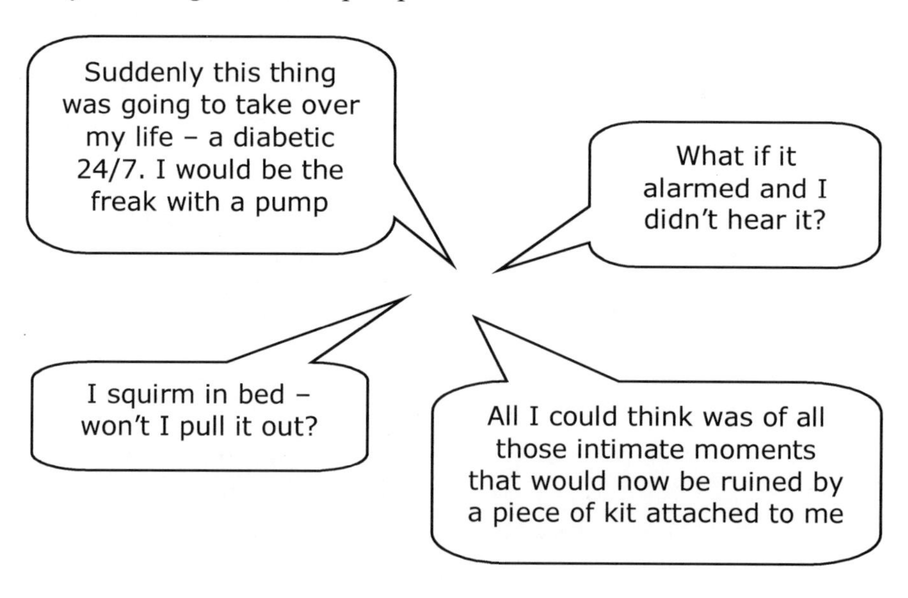

The overall picture

Table 1: Summary of the pros and cons of pump therapy

Positive aspects	Negative aspects
* No more injections * Insulin works more predictably * Feeling more successful and confident * Improved HbA1c levels * Less planning ahead * Easier to manage physical activity * Eat what you want, when you want	* Wearing the pump 24/7 * Hard work * Insecurity * No days off * What if it doesn't work for me? * Affecting your whole life?

The information in this section may have given you food for thought, and may have brought up aspects you hadn't previously considered. The important thing to remember is that if you are considering a pump, it is your own beliefs, concerns and feelings that matter the most. Discussing these openly with your diabetes team, and not feeling pressured in either direction, will help you make the decision that will work the best for you.

Chapter 2: Getting your pump

If you like what you've read so far, and want to see if you can get an insulin pump, this chapter will take you through the next steps.

Discussions with your diabetes team

The first step to success is to have a discussion about your diabetes with your diabetes team, and find out their thoughts about you using an insulin pump. Many health professionals are very positive about using insulin pumps, and it may have been something they were already thinking about. Other health professionals have less knowledge about pump therapy and may not be experienced in using them, so they may need to find out more before having further conversations with you about it.

If they agree with your idea, they will want to do a proper assessment (see pages 27 to 29) and then they will be able to give you an appointment to start using a pump or you may go on a waiting list for a short period of time.

If your enquiries are generally met with support but there are reasons why your health professional feels that it is not yet the right option, you may be asked to undertake various tasks, for example:

- Attending a structured education course to learn more about diabetes, intensive management and carbohydrate counting – this type of course is a standard pre-pump requirement in many locations
- Monitoring your blood glucose more often, and working closely with your diabetes team to see if your diabetes control can be improved in other ways
- Changing your insulin regimen, particularly if you are not yet using analogue insulins, which may potentially improve your blood glucose levels

When you have done whichever of the above options apply to you, you can then have further discussions with your health professional about starting pump therapy, if you still feel it is an option you would like to try.

You may find that your health professional is less supportive, which could be for a number of reasons:

* They are less familiar with pump therapy in general and have reservations about using it because of their lack of knowledge and experience
* They have previously experienced (or heard about problems with) the early, less reliable insulin pumps of the 1970s and 1980s
* They have specific reasons why they feel a pump is not for you

Whatever the reason, if you are being discouraged but feel you want to persevere, there are a number of places you can go to find out more information. This will then mean that you can have more informed and constructive discussions with your diabetes team.

Other information and support

The following organisations and websites will provide you with information about the current availability of insulin pumps, how to go about getting one if you are encountering difficulties, and where you can talk to other pump users.

NICE

NICE, the National Institute for Health and Clinical Excellence, assesses treatments that are new to the NHS in England and Wales, including medication and technology such as insulin pumps. They have a team of experts for the particular clinical area focused on, and also a team of experts on how the new treatment fits with other NHS priorities and funding and they provide guidance to the NHS for its use. They identify the situations where an insulin pump is recommended, and it is mandatory that health professionals follow their recommendations. You can access the full guidance about insulin pumps on the Internet at www.nice.org.uk/ta151.

In summary, the main criteria for being suitable for a pump for adults and children over the age of 12 are:

either

* that trying to reach your target HbA1c level means you suffer from disabling hypoglycaemia, which is classed as repeated and unpredictable hypoglycaemia which causes persistent anxiety about when it will happen again, and therefore affects your quality of life

  or

* you have an HbA1c of 8.5% or above even though you are already using multiple daily injections, including using long-acting insulin analogues

In addition, if you start to use a pump, NICE guidance says that you should only continue to use it if the initial improvements are sustained, so as long as you either have a better HbA1c level or you have less unpredictable hypoglycaemia, you can continue using your pump.

For children under 12, the rules are slightly different. An insulin pump can be used if multiple daily injections are thought to be impractical or inappropriate. If young children start pump therapy without a trial of multiple daily injections, NICE guidance states that they should then try multiple daily injections between the ages of 12 and 18, because otherwise, they won't have had any experience of whether they prefer that to using a pump or find that it suits their diabetes better.

INPUT

INPUT (INsulin PUmp Therapy) is an organisation set up by people with diabetes to help people have access to insulin pump therapy if they want to use a pump and might benefit from using one. Its focus is on Type 1 diabetes, but the organisation hopes eventually to also help people with Type 2 diabetes access pump therapy.

INPUT works with the Department of Health and other organisations to help improve understanding of insulin pump therapy and how it can help people with diabetes. If you have difficulty getting an insulin pump because your local health care commissioning organisation does not support them financially, INPUT can help you put a case together. All the information you need is on their website at www.input.me.uk, and they are happy to be contacted by individuals.

Pump manufacturers

The websites of the pump manufacturing companies provide information on the benefits of their particular insulin pumps, but they also can provide a lot of objective information about the ways that pumps can help with diabetes management. INPUT's website, detailed above, provides an up to date list of the pump companies in the UK and links to their websites.

Diabetes UK

Diabetes UK supports the appropriate use of insulin pump therapy according to "clinical need, personal choice and suitability". You can view Diabetes UK's position statement, which outlines their support for pumps, on their website at www.diabetes.org.uk/pumps. As with INPUT, Diabetes UK works with the Department of Health and other organisations to ensure that people are assessed for using pump therapy on the basis of need rather than availability of local funding.

Talking to other pump users

The main Internet forum for talking to others in the UK is www.insulin-pumpers.org.uk, where you can read about other people's experiences, talk to them and have your questions answered. There are also many other forums and blogs that you can access, including www.diabetessupport.co.uk which has a specific forum for pump users.

You may also have the opportunity to talk directly to other pump users in your area – ask your diabetes team if there is any formal way of this happening, for example a support group or discussion forum, or otherwise ask if you can be put in touch with other local pump users.

Successful Diabetes Tip

The more you can find out about pump therapy before you start, particularly by talking to people already using pumps, will mean you will ensure you are well prepared for your life with a pump.

Where to next?

The information you have found out from these and other sources may reinforce your decision to try and get a pump, or may result in you deciding that you don't want to go ahead. If you decide to persevere, you may need to make a special case to your health care commissioning organisation, or satisfy your health professional team that you are able to manage a pump. Equally, if you decide not to persevere, it's important to realise that you can always rethink your decision at a later date or if there comes a time when you feel your diabetes will be easier to manage using an insulin pump.

Assessments before starting to use your pump

Whilst some assessments you have will vary according to the organisation of your local diabetes service and their expertise in pump therapy, there are a number of aspects that are commonly looked at before starting pump therapy:

Your HbA1c

As described in the NICE section of this ebook (see page 23), there are national criteria that determine whether your HbA1c level suggests a pump will be useful to you. However, this is not the only factor, so if you have a lower HbA1c than the guidance states, this does not necessarily mean that you won't be able to get a pump.

Hypoglycaemia

The amount and type of hypoglycaemia you have is important – frequent hypoglycaemia, particularly with no warning, or wide swings in your blood glucose level that seem to be impossible to sort out, can indicate that you would benefit from pump therapy.

Your insulin regimen

In most circumstances, you will be encouraged to make sure your insulin regimen is the best it can be to help you get your diabetes under control before pump therapy will be considered.

Insulin analogues (see Table 2) give you the flexibility to match your insulin doses more closely to your food and daily activities. If you are using an insulin regimen which includes pre-mixed insulins, or which includes isophane insulin once or twice a day, you may be asked to try out using analogue insulins before being considered for a pump.

Table 2: Insulin analogues

Basal (long acting) analogues	Bolus (rapid acting) analogues
Lantus (insulin glargine) Levemir (insulin detemir)	Humalog (insulin lispro) Novorapid (insulin aspart) Apidra (insulin glulisine)

Your injection sites

Lumpy injection sites, or lipohypertrophy, are a common cause of swinging blood glucose levels, because the way that insulin is absorbed from a lumpy site is very unpredictable, so it may work fast one day and hardly at all another day. If you have lumpy injection sites, you will probably be asked to completely avoid injecting into them before you are considered for pump therapy. As with the insulin regimen changes above, this is to try and get the best blood glucose control you can and may mean that you don't need a pump if you can obtain this control by other means.

Emotional coping

This is an important aspect, as there may be many reasons why using a pump might give you unacceptable stress and anxiety, including:

- Being concerned about having a pump attached to you (as discussed on page 17 and pages 45 to 46)
- Feeling like your diabetes is on show to others, rather than something that can be kept to yourself
- Whether it will affect close relationships, particularly if you are just getting to know someone
- Feeling under pressure to obtain good blood glucose results
- Feeling like a pump is a last resort and it **has** to work

If any of these apply to you, it is important that the pros and cons of using a pump are very carefully discussed before you go ahead. For some people, there are no psychological issues at all; for others, they play a major part and might be the primary reason for continuing with injections rather than using a pump. You might feel some apprehension but want to go ahead, but if you then find that when you start using a pump you experience huge anxiety and feel distressed, talk to your health professional and consider whether you would prefer to start using injections again instead.

Your commitment

This is often referred to as 'motivation', and includes your willingness to undertake multiple blood glucose tests each day, actively adjust your insulin doses, and generally take a proactive approach to managing your diabetes. If you have felt that none of your efforts with your diabetes have worked in the past, you may have reduced your testing frequency and stopped adjusting your insulin doses because nothing seems to work. Having open and honest discussions with your health professional can help to establish whether you are committed to working hard at your diabetes. An insulin pump cannot do the work for you, and if you wanted a pump because you felt it would be an easier option, this type of therapy probably isn't for you.

Capability

It is important that you (or your carer if they are involved in helping you manage your diabetes) have the capability to manage an insulin pump. This includes both physical and cognitive ability to work the pump. If there are physical difficulties in using the pump, for example if you have limited eyesight but have a strong support network where others could help with filling the tube and ensuring there are no air bubbles, you may be able to manage a pump using the audible beeps it gives.

Cognitive ability in this instance means the ability to make the day to day decisions required to use a pump. This doesn't mean you need to be a mathematician (although it can help!!), but you need to be able to confidently identify what insulin doses you need, when those doses should be increased or decreased, and be able to give the doses you need. There are many sources of help to calculate insulin doses, and many insulin pumps have built-in calculators to help with this, but the ultimate responsibility lies with you, and your health professional has a duty to ensure that you can use a pump safely.

General preparation

Prior to starting insulin pump therapy, making sure that you are prepared is likely to reduce your anxiety about trying something new, and help you still feel you have control over what happens to your diabetes. There are a number of aspects that you can deal with in advance, and also some specific preparations that need to be made for the actual day you start using your pump.

Carbohydrate counting

You will probably be expected to attend a local course to help you learn more about matching insulin doses to the carbohydrate you eat. The most common course is DAFNE (Dose Adjustment For Normal Eating), but there are many other types of courses around the country based on similar principles. Or you may simply have individual appointments with a specialist diabetes dietitian to help you learn about carbohydrate counting. There are also some excellent online and printed resources available to help you, such as BDEC (www.bdec-e-learning.com) and Carbs and Cals (www.carbsandcals.com).

Whatever method is used, being confident about how much carbohydrate you are eating, and how quickly it will break down into glucose in your bloodstream, are the first steps to identifying how much insulin you need to avoid unnecessary variations in your blood glucose level. If you feel you do not know enough about assessing the carbohydrate content of the different foods you eat, talk to your health professional about what is available locally to help you learn, and you can also access the additional resources already mentioned.

Successful Diabetes Tip

Feeling experienced and confident in assessing the amount and type of carbohydrate in your food before you start using an insulin pump will take some of the stress out of learning a new way of managing your diabetes.

Choosing your insulin pump

There are an increasing number of insulin pumps available, incorporating sophisticated technology. It can be difficult, or even impossible, to make an objective assessment of the whole range of insulin pumps available, and you are likely to find that your health professionals use a limited number of models. Websites such as www.insulin-pumpers.org.uk and www.input.me.uk, both run by people who are passionate about helping others access insulin pump therapy, can provide objective information about different pumps and also opportunities to ask questions and talk to other pump users to find out their experiences of using different pumps. It is worth keeping in mind that all insulin pumps are extremely accurate and reliable with multiple built-in safety systems, and are also becoming much easier to use than in the past. Your choice of pump might be influenced by the following:

- The size of the pump
- What the pump looks like
- How the pump can integrate with your blood glucose meter and use the results to help you make decisions about your insulin doses
- What personal information the pump can store, such as your usual insulin to carbohydrate ratios, your correction doses, or a library of the carbohydrate values of foods you regularly eat
- The ability of the pump to calculate insulin doses for you to reduce the potential for making a mistake
- The availability of computer software to be able to analyse your blood glucose control over longer periods of time
- The ability for your pump information to be shared with health professionals electronically to help you make the most of your own pump management

Talking to your health professionals about the different features of the available pumps, as well as talking to other pump users if you can, will help you decide how they might benefit you.

Help and support you can expect

Before you start

As already discussed, to start using a pump you will be expected to work closely with your health professional, to carry out the assessments described earlier in this chapter and then to move forward and start pump therapy. If you are able to meet with other pump users, that can be invaluable, and might be a standard part of the process of getting a pump from your diabetes team.

The other aspect of preparation that is helpful is to be able to look at and physically handle an insulin pump before you start using it. You might be able to borrow one for a few days from your diabetes team, or have the opportunity in clinic to spend some time handling a pump. Some clinics have the full range of insulin pumps available; others may use one or two but be able to get hold of others for you if you want them to. All insulin pumps are reliable, but vary in their set-up, functions and the way you programme them.

Your pre-pump support should include information about when you will start pump therapy – how long your appointment will be (it is common to spend a few hours at that first appointment), whether it will be with others or an individual appointment. In many diabetes teams, people new to using pumps have the opportunity to learn together in groups. This can be really valuable, as it helps you feel less alone, and also you can swap stories and learn from each other as well as getting the answers to many of your questions. In other areas, possibly because of the number of pump users or the organisation of the service, you may have an individual appointment.

Planning for the big day

Prior to the day you start your pump, your diabetes team should also help you to identify how best to reduce your insulin so that you don't have the pump insulin and your usual insulin working at the same time. This usually involves cutting down on your longer-acting insulin, although you may still have some of this working in the first day or two of using a pump. You should also have a realistic idea of what will happen on your 'pump start day', so that you can plan your food intake and your insulin injections around this.

Once you are using your pump

Once you have started pump therapy, you should expect to have fairly close contact with, and, easy access to your diabetes team. Some diabetes teams (and some pump manufacturing companies) offer 24 hour helplines, but in any case, regular appointments and telephone or email contact in the first few weeks is the norm.

> Initially you have a lot of questions and need a great deal of support, both face to face and on the phone

Chapter 3: Getting started with your pump

After all the preparation and learning, once you've got that long-awaited start date, you'll need to make some practical adjustments to make your pump start go as smoothly as possible. This chapter focuses on the preparation immediately beforehand and on setting your initial insulin pump doses. This, chapter, together with chapter 4, 'early days with your pump', will give you the basic information you need to deal with the first few days of using your pump. Your health professional will offer guidance on all the aspects discussed here, as there are likely to be local variation in both the systems that are in place and in the advice given.

Long acting insulin adjustment pre-pump

When you use injection therapy, this includes injections of longer- and shorter-acting insulin, which may be pre-mixed or may be taken by you at different times of the day. This is because you need a supply of insulin 24 hours a day, ie between the times you inject, as well as needing additional insulin when you eat food that contains carbohydrate.

When you use an insulin pump, you no longer take any longer-acting insulin, because the pump will give you a constant supply of rapid-acting insulin 24 hours a day. This makes it much easier for you to respond quickly to variations in your lifestyle and your blood glucose levels, and also takes away some of the uncertainty of how much active insulin you currently have in your bloodstream.

For the first day or two of using your insulin pump, you are likely to still have some longer-acting insulin in your body, and you will also be having a continuous supply of rapid-acting insulin through your pump. These two insulins will overlap and so can increase the chances of you having a hypo. To reduce the risk of this happening, the longer-acting insulin you take in the 24 hours leading up to your pump start should be reduced. How this should be achieved will vary according to your individual insulin regimen, but as a general guide, your most recent dose should be reduced by around 50%, and in some cases, if the timing of the pump start is quite close to the time you would have taken your longer-acting insulin, you may be asked to omit that dose completely.

Your shorter-acting insulin may also need to be reduced, to avoid your last dose overlapping with the initial doses from your pump. Your health professional will work with you to make a plan that will work with your individual insulin regimen.

Deciding on your blood glucose targets

When you start to use an insulin pump, deciding what blood glucose level you will be aiming for will help you make decisions about your insulin doses on a daily basis. You may be used to keeping your blood glucose level high to avoid suddenly dipping into hypos, or you may be keen to get your blood glucose as tightly controlled as you possibly can.

Working with your health professional to identify your initial target doses is the safest way to enjoy a smooth transition to pump therapy. If you have already started to develop long-term complications and you drop your blood glucose level too quickly, this could make the complications worsen. Also, the main aim in the early days of pump therapy is to avoid hypoglycaemia, and to try and achieve some stability in your blood glucose levels, rather than achieve the longer-term blood glucose levels you may wish for. So for example, if you have been experiencing blood glucose fluctuations of between two and 20 millimoles per litre (mmol/l), your initial target might be something like 8-14 mmol/l. Once your blood glucose is more stable, you can then start to lower the target range over a period of a few weeks.

Successful Diabetes Tip

Your initial blood glucose target range is aimed at stabilising your blood glucose level and avoiding hypos rather than aiming for perfect control. Over time, you can tighten your control as you become more confident about using your pump.

Setting your initial insulin doses

Working out what insulin doses to programme into your pump includes the continuous infusion rate (known as the **basal rate**) and also the amount of insulin to take when you eat carbohydrate (a **food bolus**) or if you have a high blood glucose level (a **correction bolus**).

Your health professional will help you to work out what initial programming to use with your pump, but if you want to work this out yourself, you can follow the guidance here.

Your basal rate

First, to work out your basal rate, identify what the average amount of insulin you need in total on a daily basis whilst you are still taking injections. If you are already altering your insulin doses to match the carbohydrate you eat, or if you regularly make changes to your insulin doses, you may need to look at a number of days to work out an average amount.

Once you have this figure, you then need to deduct a percentage – this is partly because whenever you change your insulin regimen it is always wise to be cautious about doses, and it is easier to run your blood glucose a little higher and then add insulin in than it is to deal with hypos when you are trying to find out what doses work for you. Also, you are likely to need less insulin in general as a continuous infusion tends to improve your insulin sensitivity. A reduction of around 30% of your total dose is probably sufficient, but if you are having a lot of hypos, then reducing this by either 35% or 40% is more realistic.

The amount you now have should be divided by 2 – so half of it can be given as your basal rate, and that amount will then be topped up by boluses through the day.

After dividing by 2, divide the remaining amount again, this time by 24, which will then give you an hourly rate. It is generally recommended that no more than one unit per hour is used as a starting dose, even if you have been on a much higher daily amount, because your insulin sensitivity is likely to improve using a pump, and you will need less insulin.

It is extremely unlikely that the same rate for every hour (or every half hour depending on how your pump is programmed) will be right for you, but it is simply a starting point and the individual rates for different hours can then be increased or decreased as required. How to do this is discussed on pages 61 to 62.

When you are calculating your starting basal rate, it is safer to round the numbers down, ie to calculate slightly lower doses, to make sure that you avoid hypos. Examples of how you can calculate your initial basal rate can be seen in Table 3.

Table 3: Examples of calculating your initial basal rate settings

Average total daily insulin dose	90	80	60	35
Having hypos?	No (-30%)	Yes (-40%)	No (-30%)	Yes (-40%)
After % reduction	63	48	42	21
Divided by 2	31.5	24	21	10.5
Divided by 24	1.312	0.1	0.875	0.437
Hourly rate (up to 1 unit)	**1 unit**	**0.8 units**	**1 unit**	**0.4 units**

Your food boluses

Food boluses are doses of insulin that are taken in relation to the carbohydrate you eat, which are calculated using your **insulin to carbohydrate ratio**, ie how much insulin you need for a certain amount of carbohydrate.

The way you calculate your insulin to carbohydrate ratio may be slightly different from when you had injections, because you may have been adding extra insulin to match any snacks you have between meals, but when you use your pump, because you can give additional insulin at any time without an extra injection, you only give insulin for the food that you are definitely going to eat at that particular moment.

So if you have a plate of food but think you might only be able to eat half of it, you can give insulin for that amount of food and then top it up at the end of the meal if you have eaten more than you expected to. Similarly, if you are eating a main course but are unsure if you will have a dessert, you can give insulin just for the main course and add another dose if you decide to have a dessert. This flexibility is one of the main bonuses of an insulin pump, because it means that you don't have to take extra insulin 'just in case' and you also don't have to eat extra food because you have got more insulin than you need in your body.

If you are already calculating how much insulin to take at mealtimes according to the amount of carbohydrate in your meals, you can use this ratio as a starting point for your pump. You may find that your insulin requirements reduce when you use a pump instead of injections, in which case you can reduce your ratio if you find that your existing one is too high.

If you haven't already learnt what your usual insulin to carbohydrate ratio is, you can do one of two things:

1. Use a standard ratio as a starting point, such as one unit of insulin to 10 grams of carbohydrate, which is a method that many specialist diabetes teams use. Or if your insulin requirements have been particularly small, or for children, you may use a lower amount of insulin such as one unit of insulin to 20 grams of carbohydrate.

2. The second option is to use what is known as the '500 rule', which was determined by clinical experience and uses your pre-pump insulin doses. To use this calculation, take the total amount of insulin you needed pre-pump on average over a 24

hour period, reduce it by 30% or 40% as detailed in the previous section, then divide 500 by your total. See Table 4 for how this works in practice – the units have been rounded up or down to make the calculations easier. As you will see, the results are relatively close to 1 unit to 10g of carbohydrate, except where the total daily dose is much smaller, so one unit of insulin will be enough for a greater amount of carbohydrate.

Table 4: Using the 500 rule to calculate your insulin to carbohydrate ratio

Average total daily insulin dose	90	80	60	35
Having hypos?	No (-30%)	Yes (-40%)	No (-30%)	Yes (-40%)
After % reduction	63	48	42	21
Divided 500 by total	500/63 = 7.9	500/48 =10.4	500/42 = 11.9	500/21 = 23.8
1 unit of insulin to:	**8g CHO**	**10g CHO**	**9g CHO**	**25g CHO**

Neither of these methods are superior to the other, mainly because if the reason you are starting to use a pump is because you have difficulty controlling your blood glucose levels, then your usual daily insulin dose is not going to be an accurate guide to how much insulin you will actually need using a pump. Also, your sensitivity to insulin is likely to increase. And thirdly, you won't be able to accurately judge whether your insulin to carbohydrate ratio is working until you have got rid of the longer-acting insulin in your body, so selecting a dose simply as a starting point makes sense.

You may find that calculating your ratio using the 500 rule, and comparing it with the initial starting ratio that you have decided upon, lets you know if the dose is likely to be in the right area. You can find information on how to assess and adjust your insulin to carbohydrate ratio on page 63.

Type and timing of your food boluses

As well as deciding how much insulin you need, you also need to decide how quickly you need it. The standard bolus function on your pump is the simplest to use, and gives you the whole dose of insulin within a few seconds, the same as the injections you used before getting your pump. And many insulin pumps can calculate the amounts for you, so all you then have to do is press a button to activate it.

If you are eating a sweet snack or something containing less than 50 grams of carbohydrate, giving the bolus immediately is fine. This can be just before you eat, whilst you are eating, or immediately after you have eaten. For meals which contain large amounts of carbohydrate, or are higher in protein or fat, the glucose will be released more slowly into your bloodstream, and so a bolus which matches this release will be more effective at keeping your blood glucose well-balanced.

Your pump will also give you a number of other options of how you can give a bolus, such as extending the insulin delivery over a longer period, or giving some insulin immediately and some over a longer period or as a separate dose. More information about these types of boluses can be found on pages 64 to 65.

Your correction boluses

Correction boluses are the extra doses of insulin that you take if your blood glucose is out of your target range. As with your food boluses, as you get used to your pump you will recognise what correction bolus ratio works for you, which is how much your blood glucose will reduce by each unit of insulin you take.

There are two methods of choosing a starting point:

1. Using a standard ratio of one unit of insulin for every 2.5 mmol/l that you want your blood glucose to drop.

2. Using the '100 rule', where you divide 100 by the total daily dose of insulin (minus the 30% or 40% as before), as shown in Table 5.

Table 5: Using the 100 rule to calculate your insulin to blood glucose correction ratio

Average total daily insulin dose	90	80	60	35
Having hypos?	No (-30%)	Yes (-40%)	No (-30%)	Yes (-40%)
After % reduction	63	48	42	21
Divided 100 by total	100/63 = 1.58	100/48 = 2.08	100/42 = 2.38	100/21 = 4.76
1 unit of insulin will lower your blood glucose by:	**1.5 mmol/l**	**2 mmol/l**	**2.5 mmol/l**	**5 mmol/l**

When you were taking insulin injections, you may simply have increased the amount of insulin you were giving with your next meal to correct your blood glucose. The advantage of using an insulin pump is that you can take an extra bolus at any point. This means that you can spend much less time with your blood glucose outside your target range, which can help you feel more energised and also increase your protection against long-term complications. Correction boluses should not be taken more frequently than two hourly intervals, as the previous bolus will not have finished working.

In addition to previous correction doses, it is also important to take account of other things that have been happening in the past few hours that affect your blood glucose level, and also what you are about to do, before you decide to take a correction bolus. The factors to account for are:

* When you last ate – if you have eaten some food which contains carbohydrate in the last two hours, your blood glucose may not have returned to the level you would expect. You should therefore wait the full two hours after you have eaten before you correct a high blood glucose reading.
* When you last gave yourself an insulin dose – this applies both to food boluses and previous correction doses. In both cases, you should wait two hours since your last insulin dose before correcting a high reading. Some insulin pumps have an 'insulin on board' function, which gives you an indication of how much of your last insulin bolus is still to be used up.
* Whether you are about to be physically active or do something else that might lower your blood glucose in the next few hours.

If you have not given any insulin or eaten in the last two hours, and you are not anticipating doing anything to further lower your blood glucose, then you would give a correction dose. To work out how much to give, work out how many millimoles per litre you want your blood glucose to drop, and then use your correction ratio to work out how much insulin to give. So for example:

Current blood glucose = 14 mmol/l

Target range = 7-10 mmol/l

Amount you want your blood glucose to drop = 4-7 mmol/l

Correction ratio = 1 unit to 2 mmol/l

Amount of insulin to take = 2 or 3 units

You may be able to use your insulin pump to do the calculations for you, if your pump has that feature. For this, you programme in advance your usual correction ratio and your target blood glucose range, and make sure the pump has the information about your blood glucose level, and the pump will provide a suggestion of how much insulin you need. However, the pump will not give you the bolus until you have agreed to it, so you still need to take action.

If you are unwell, you may find that you need to correct your blood glucose every two hours, and also increase your basal rate, to keep pace with the amount of insulin your body needs to cope with the raised blood glucose that is likely to occur as a result of being unwell. Pages 74-75 provide detailed information on how to deal with illness.

Successful Diabetes Tip

Testing your blood glucose frequently and correcting high blood glucose levels when they appear can help you be more in control of your diabetes and reduce your risk of long-term complications

Chapter 4: Early days with your pump

This chapter focuses on the early days of getting used to your pump, and dealing with the aspects you are most likely to encounter. There is also more information about living with your pump in chapter 7, which you can refer to later, although depending on your day to day life, some of that information may also need to be accessed during the early days.

Wearing your pump

When you get your pump, you will also receive one or two pouches or clips to hold it. You can obtain other holders from your pump manufacturer, and also websites such as those listed in Table 6 provide alternative holders including backpacks, belts and t-shirts with pouches, many designed particularly with small children in mind.

Table 6: Pump holder websites

www.angelbearpumpwear.com
www.insulinpumpfashions.com
www.myownstylepack.com
www.pumpwearinc.com
www.insulinpumppacksforyou.com

The easiest places to wear your pump are:

* In your trouser or shirt pocket
* Clipped to your waistband
* Strapped to your arm or leg under clothing
* If female: tucked into your bra or attached under your arm to your bra
* In your pyjama pockets
* In pouches sewn into your clothing

If your pump can be operated with a wireless device, you will be able to give boluses and make changes to your infusion rates with your pump still tucked securely and discreetly away, which might influence where you decide to wear it. It is also important to make sure that if your pump has a length of tubing between the pump and the infusion site, this needs to be tucked away, otherwise it can easily get caught on door handles and other objects. The pump also needs to be secured especially well if you are undertaking any strenuous sports, unless you choose to disconnect your pump for a short while, which is discussed on pages 72 to 74.

If you have a pump attached with tubing, you may be concerned about where you can put your insulin pump during the night, and whether you will accidentally give extra insulin whilst you are asleep. It is fine to leave the pump loose in your bed, or tucked under your pillow, and the safety features of the pump mean that you won't accidentally give extra insulin during the night. Also, if you are female, you may find it easier to wear clothing which splits at the waist rather than dresses, to enable you to access your pump at any time.

Dealing with the psychological effects

You may have been apprehensive about starting to use an insulin pump, particularly if you believe that it is a sort of 'last chance' to sort your diabetes out. Or you may not have thought that it would have any negative aspects, but once you have the pump, you feel quite negative towards it even if you hadn't expected to.

The most common concerns raised by people starting to use an insulin pump include:

- Feeling like a beginner again – although you may be going onto a pump because your diabetes hasn't been perfectly controlled in the past, you will have had routines and ways of dealing with the highs and lows you experience. Because your insulin is being delivered in a completely different way, starting out with a pump can feel like starting to learn about diabetes all over again

* Concerns that you may not be able to achieve what you want to achieve in terms of stability of your glucose levels
* A feeling of your diabetes being 'on show', whereas before it was simply a matter of discreetly giving injections
* The pump constantly reminding you about your diabetes, rather than something you didn't like to think about as often
* Worries about close relationships – how will your partner, children and family cope with it, or how you might introduce the topic if starting a new relationship

Whatever the reason, talking to someone about your feelings – your health professionals, your friends and family, or other pump users – will help you to deal with any negative feelings. If you feel very strongly, this may be a reason to stop using your pump and revert back to injection therapy. If you choose this option, keep in mind that it is an entirely reasonable decision to make and you should not feel guilty or that you have failed, and of course you can always try the pump again if you decide it will work for you in the future.

If your feelings are less strong, you may want to persevere with the pump, particularly if you start to see benefits with your blood glucose levels, but it is still worth talking to someone about the way you feel and to seek additional help or support if you feel you need it. This additional support may come from your local health professionals or may come from other pump users, who will have the added benefit of going through situations and possibly feelings similar to your own.

Blood glucose testing

Checking your blood glucose levels is an essential part of being able to successfully manage your pump, to be able to assess how well your insulin doses are controlling your blood glucose level. Frequent testing at the start of your 'pump journey' will give you information about the accuracy of your basal rate, your insulin to carbohydrate ratio, your correction ratio, and also how your blood glucose alters in different situations.

As a minimum, it is recommended that you test at least seven times a day when you first start using your pump, as shown in table 7.

Table 7: Recommended minimum blood glucose testing when starting out with a pump

When to test	What you can use the results for
Before breakfast, lunch and evening meal	To identify whether your basal rate is set correctly in the hours leading up to this time. To provide a starting point to assess the effectiveness of your meal dose. To help you make decisions about the dose of insulin to take before your meal, ie if you need to add any units to correct a high reading or take less if you are close to a hypo.
2 hours after breakfast, lunch and evening meal	To check whether your bolus insulin you took for your meal was the right dose.
Before bed	To identify whether your basal rate is set correctly in the hours leading up to this time and also make decisions about any insulin dose changes you need to make before bed.

There are also a number of other times when testing can be useful when you are using pump therapy, as follows:

- 2-3 am: roughly the midpoint of the night, so you can assess your basal rate for the hours before and after
- 2 hours after you have taken a correction dose
- 2 hours after changing your infusion site to ensure that the insulin is infusing properly
- At 2-3 hour intervals **without** eating carbohydrates, to assess your basal rate (see pages 61-62 for more information on this)

The times that anyone with diabetes might carry out additional blood glucose tests also apply, for example if you are undertaking physical activity, drinking alcohol, are unwell, before driving, or if you suspect you are hypo (see pages 57-59 for more information on hypos).

As you become more confident with your pump, you may choose to adopt a different pattern of blood glucose testing. If you manage to reduce the swings in your blood glucose levels, you may also find that you become more aware of even small fluctuations in your blood glucose, and testing to confirm whether your awareness is correct will help you learn even more about managing your diabetes successfully.

People who have had pumps for a few years say they still test relatively frequently, as they find it helps them make their insulin dose decisions and also provides reassurance that they are within their target range.

Caring for your infusion sites

The recommended sites for inserting your cannula are:

* Your abdomen, either above or below your belly button
* The upper outer parts of your buttocks
* The middle and outer side of your thighs

Some people use the upper part of their arms as well, but this is not recommended as the layer of subcutaneous fat on your upper arms is very thin, so the cannula may infuse insulin into your muscle, which will make it absorb very erratically and make it more difficult for you to control your blood glucose level.

It is important to ensure that you do not site the cannula in any areas where you already have lipohypertrophy (lumps from previously injecting there frequently), as this will affect the absorption of your insulin. Also, ensuring that the cannula is at least two centimetres away from your belly button or from any scars will help to ensure good absorption of your insulin.

Prior to inserting your cannula, washing your hands and ensuring that the infusion site is clean and dry is important, to avoid infections at the infusion site. If you find that you are prone to infusion site infections, you may need to use some additional type of disinfection such as antiseptic wipes – your health professional will advise you on the most suitable types.

Some cannulae have insertion devices, either reusable or disposable, which can make life easier. In all cases, following the manufacturer's advice on how to insert the cannula will make the procedure easier.

The cannula should be changed every two to three days, and with experience you will learn what works best for you. If you find that your blood glucose levels remain stable, every three days is fine, but if you notice that your blood glucose level starts to rise on the third day, it is an indication that changing it after two days will suit you better. If you leave the cannula in longer than the recommended time, this not only might affect your insulin absorption, but more importantly will give you a high risk of infection. Any infection is likely to need treatment with antibiotics to prevent a more serious abscess, so seek medical help from your GP or your insulin pump team if you suspect your site may have become infected.

If you change the infusion tubing as well, it is important to remember to prime the tubing by filling it with insulin before connecting to your body. Also some cannula manufacturers recommend that you give a bolus of 0.5 units of insulin when you first attach it, to fill the space in the cannula when the needle is removed – check the specific instructions with your equipment to find out if you need to do this.

You may need to change your cannula more frequently at times. For example, if you notice any redness at the infusion site, or if your site becomes uncomfortable before it is due to be changed. If in doubt, it is safer to change more frequently. When you first insert the cannula you may experience some discomfort, but this should disappear within two hours. If your infusion site is still painful after this time, it is unlikely to settle and you will need to insert a new cannula in a different site.

Testing your blood glucose two hours after changing your infusion site is recommended, to check that your insulin is infusing properly. This means that you might need to think carefully about when you change your site for example, changing just before you go to bed will be less practical than changing the site during the day.

Successful Diabetes Tip

Making sure you change your cannula every 2-3 days means that your insulin can be properly absorbed and greatly reduces your risk of infection at your infusion site

Record Keeping

All insulin pumps have memories where data are collected about any information you programme into the pump, plus data which are stored automatically such as the insulin doses you have given. This data can be downloaded into a computer or other electronic device, or some pumps will download automatically at set intervals. You may choose to use your downloaded data to make decisions about your insulin doses, you may choose to keep handwritten records, or you may choose to simply use the information that is stored in your pump. There are pros and cons to each of these methods, as this section will describe.

Computer download records

The most useful aspect of using downloaded data is being able to look at many different aspects of your results relatively quickly. This includes your blood glucose readings, your insulin doses, the amount of carbohydrate you have been eating, and other lifestyle factors such as physical activity. You choose how much information you need to store to be able to get the most out of your data.

You can look at a lot of the data in detail, such as individual days, trends over longer periods of time, particular times of the day in detail, and much more. You can also choose the type of data that are most useful to you, for example a graph or chart may be easier to interpret than a list of numbers.

It can take time to work out which data help you the most and how to analyse all your results, but over time, the rewards include being able to proactively adjust your insulin doses rather than just reacting to individual readings. Your health professional can help you interpret the data and make sense of it.

Written records

Manually writing down your records gives you the option of recording your information in the most useful way to you, such as the varying severity of any hypoglycaemia you experience, or how accurate you believe your carbohydrate estimation to be. The information can be easily referred back at any point, including many years later, for example if you want to find information about previous insulin doses or how you coped when you flew across time zones.

You can also use a computer-generated spreadsheet if you want to look at trends in your insulin doses etc, although that might be slightly harder to do if you use written records.

Pump-held records

Using only the information your pump stores is probably the simplest way of looking at your records, and you always have that data to hand in your pump. However, it is likely to limit your ability to look back at trends and may mean that you manage your pump insulin doses more reactively, but as technology increases, it is likely that more information will be available through your pump and that you will be able to look at past results and trends without always referring to downloaded data.

Useful information to record

This section looks at the type of information you might find useful to keep, and why. It is easy to believe that you can rely on your memory, but the varying information you might find useful means that recording it is the only way you can look at everything. You may not need all this information every day, but depending on the aspects of your diabetes you may be worried about, different information will be useful at different times. For example, if you are concerned about your blood glucose levels being inadequately controlled after meals, then the information suggested in the 'food and drink' and 'insulin boluses you have taken' sections that follow will be useful to you.

Your blood glucose levels

Your blood glucose readings are a key part of being able to manage your pump therapy. In addition to the numbers themselves, noting what they relate to can be helpful – for example were you testing to find out the effect of specific types or amounts of food or drink, or to monitor how physical activity has affected your blood glucose level. Keeping a note of these aspects will give you information to help make sense of why your levels have risen or fallen, and also help you manage similar situations even better in the future.

Food and drink

When recording your food and drink, this includes not only the amount of carbohydrate but also the type of food, to assist in identifying the amount of fat or protein, and whether the combination of foods has a high or low glycaemic index, all of which influence the length of time your blood glucose may be affected. Experimenting with different bolus doses can help you find the most useful ones to use for the different types of foods you like to eat.

Insulin boluses you have taken

When recording your insulin bolus doses, noting the reason for each bolus can be useful, for example whether it is to correct a high blood glucose or to match your food intake. It also makes the results more meaningful when you reflect back, as it tells you what particular aspect you are trying to remedy. The type of bolus can also be useful, for example you would expect a standard bolus to work more quickly than an extended or mixed bolus.

Temporary basal rates used

Noting the time that temporary basal rates are started and finished, as well as the amount of increase or decrease, will tell you whether it has had the desired effect on your blood glucose levels. This is particularly useful for situations that might not occur every day, such as a bout of flu.

Changes made to basal rates or to bolus ratios

Identifying the times when you made more major changes to your insulin doses, for example altering your basal rate or your food or correction bolus rates, will help you to make sense of any alterations in your blood glucose levels.

Hypoglycaemia

Include not only that you were hypo, but the cause if you know it (or the suspected cause), how low your blood glucose dropped, what symptoms you experienced and what you used to treat it.

Hyperglycaemia

As with hypoglycaemia, keep a record of your blood glucose levels, what symptoms you had, and what additional insulin you needed to take to deal with it. Also note the cause, particularly if it is something that recurs (for example during a menstrual cycle), so that next time you will be able to deal with it promptly, or even alter your insulin doses proactively to avoid it happening.

Specific situations

If you are doing something unusual, or something that is different from the rest of your day, for example going to the gym or attending a party, write down what actions you took to keep your blood glucose level within your range, and how well it worked. Again, this is information that, built up over time, will enable you to manage your diabetes much more easily and make decisions about your insulin doses that you can rely on.

Alcohol

If you are drinking alcohol, the type and amount you are drinking, including any mixer drinks, can help you identify the causes of any high or low blood glucose readings.

Removing your pump

If you take your pump off for any length of time, even if just for showering, noting how long the pump was off and how much difference the time without insulin made to your blood glucose level can help you identify if you need to take any corrective action, and also how long it is safe to keep your pump off for.

Infusion site or infusion set changes

Because the effectiveness of your insulin dose depends on how well it is absorbed, noting when you make changes can help you work out the optimum amount of time between infusion site changes. It might also identify whether you get better control of your blood glucose levels using some sites rather than others. There is also likely to be a relationship between any infusion site infections you experience and how long the infusion set has been left in.

The date and time for all records

Finally, knowing the date and the time of everything you record will help you see the relationship between the food you eat, the daily activities you undertake and the doses of insulin you are taking.

Table 8: Summary of useful information to record

* Your blood glucose levels
* Any food or drink you have consumed that contains carbohydrate
* Insulin boluses you have taken
* Temporary basal rates used
* Changes made to basal rates or to bolus ratios
* Any hypoglycaemia and what action you took
* Any hyperglycaemia and what action you took
* Specific situations that could affect your blood glucose level, eg physical activity
* Any alcohol you drank

This may seem a large amount of information to record, but it will help you see the full picture of what is going on. Over time, you may find that you record much less information, but at the beginning of your journey, it is likely to be vital to take all the influences on your blood glucose level into account.

Using Your Pump Records

As you have seen from the previous section, there is potentially a huge amount of information you can record. To help you decide what is most useful to you, keep in mind that you are simply keeping information to learn more about how you can manage your diabetes with your pump, and to help you plan ahead, particularly for recurring situations.

You may find you want to keep intensive records for relatively short periods such as when you first start using your pump, or when circumstances change in your life that are likely to affect your diabetes. Or you might prefer to record a lot of information all the time, particularly if you find it helpful. Many pump users have described the value they get out of recording their information, and how they use it to manage their pump, whereas previously when they were taking injections of insulin they found that the records were less helpful.

You may be asked to keep specific records to take along to your pump clinic. This can be valuable, as your health professional (and other pump users if you have access to group sessions) can then work with you and may have additional ideas to add to your own. Over time, small adjustments, reflection on your records and being proactive about what action to take can stop your blood glucose swings and help you to prevent situations rather than have to deal with them when they happen.

Chapter 5: Highs and Lows

This chapter focuses on high and low blood glucose readings, providing information on specific issues related to pump therapy and what you might need to do differently if you are using an insulin pump.

Hypoglycaemia

There are a number of aspects of hypoglycaemia (hypo) or a low blood glucose level that may be different when you start pump therapy. One of these is that your symptoms may change – you may start to get back some of your early warning symptoms that have been missing, such as shaking or sweating, or you may simply experience different warning symptoms. These changes usually happen because your blood glucose starts to swing less between high and low levels, and as this happens, your body starts to regain its sensitivity to insulin and your blood glucose variations reduce.

So because the warning signs you get may be altered, it becomes extremely important to test your blood glucose level whenever you suspect a hypo, as this will help you identify what blood glucose level gives you specific symptoms. Any blood glucose level below 4 mmol/l should be treated promptly before it results in a more serious drop in your blood glucose level.

Treating a hypo when you are using pump therapy becomes much easier than when using injections, mainly because you don't have any unpredictable, longer-acting insulin in your body. So any hypos you have are related to the insulin you have had in the previous few hours, rather than the insulin you may have injected many hours earlier.

The initial hypo treatment remains the same, by using fast-acting carbohydrate in the form of either a glucose drink, glucose tablets or glucose gel. But you may find that the amount of glucose you need is much smaller, mainly because your increased insulin sensitivity means you are probably experiencing the symptoms much earlier and it therefore takes less glucose to put the situation right. 10 grams of carbohydrate may be enough, or you may feel happier taking 20 grams, but it is recommended that you do not take more than this for your initial treatment.

After 10 minutes, checking your blood glucose will let you know if your treatment has started to work, and if you are still hypo at this point, a further 10 grams of fast-acting carbohydrate should be taken, and then repeat your blood glucose test another 10 minutes later.

For most people, longer-acting carbohydrates are no longer needed after the initial fast acting treatment, because any excess insulin is rapid-acting and is therefore unlikely to have a prolonged effect on your blood glucose level, unless there are unusual factors such as a prolonged reaction to physical activity or drinking alcohol, in which case you may well need some longer-acting carbohydrates. If you are in a situation where this may happen, you can proactively reduce your basal rate for a few hours following the first hypo to try and prevent it happening. Experimenting, and checking the effects on your blood glucose level, will help you grow confident about the best method of treatment for you.

Whilst it may not be necessary for everyone, you also have the option of stopping your insulin pump completely for a short period, but if you choose this option, it is recommended that you do not stop the pump for longer than 30 minutes, as this should adequately treat the hypo. Longer periods of stopping the pump are likely to result in your blood glucose rising outside your target range and can re-introduce the 'swinging' blood glucose levels that you may have experienced prior to using your pump.

Some pumps now have a built-in safety cut-out which automatically switches the pump off for a short period, and also repeats this if you do not respond, which helps to deal with hypo unawareness, particularly at night. If your pump is linked to a continuous glucose monitoring (CGM) system, it may alert you to low blood glucose readings, depending on the parameters that you have programmed into the device.

If you have a severe hypo, where you are unable to think clearly enough to treat yourself, again the pump can be stopped for a short period. Teaching your family and close friends how to either stop the pump or disconnect it means that you can avoid someone cutting the tubing in panic, as that then means you cannot reconnect without setting up a new infusion set.

Successful Diabetes Tip

Acting quickly to treat any blood glucose level lower than 4 mmol/l with rapid-acting carbohydrate will help you avoid major fluctuations in your blood glucose levels

Hyperglycaemia

Hyperglycaemia, or a high blood glucose level, becomes much more manageable when you have an insulin pump. You can give small or large correction doses at any time, and your pump may provide suggestions of what dose would be appropriate, taking into account your usual correction ratio and also any insulin from a previous bolus that might still be active. Information about how to manage correction doses can be found on pages 41 to 43.

However, because your pump only contains short-acting insulin, if for any reason your insulin delivery is interrupted, your blood glucose level can rise to a seriously high level within a few hours.

To prevent extreme rises in your blood glucose level, testing your blood glucose at key times will alert you to any significant rise so that you can treat it early. This is particularly important when you are unwell, and you'll find further information on dealing with illness on pages 74 to 76. But it is also important to test to check that insulin is being delivered effectively a couple of hours after changing your infusion set. You also then need to take action if your blood glucose is high, giving correction doses of insulin as previously discussed, to avoid ketoacidosis. The next section discusses this in more detail.

Ketoacidosis

Ketoacidosis, or DKA (Diabetic KetoAcidosis), is a condition where your body becomes acutely short of insulin. It is usually associated with illness, where increased glucose production and stress hormones combine to greatly increase the amount of insulin your body needs. But it can also be induced if you are taking much smaller amounts of insulin than your body needs, or if your insulin supply is interrupted as discussed in the previous section.

When you develop ketoacidosis, your body's shortage of insulin means that carbohydrate can't get into the cells in your body to provide them with energy. So your body starts to burn fat and muscle as an alternative source of energy, producing the waste product of ketones, which can be measured in urine and blood and can also often be smelt on your breath. The acid balance of your blood also changes and if ketoacidosis is not treated effectively, you could become seriously ill and need urgent hospital treatment.

To identify when this process starts, you should have access to some form of ketone testing, which may be for testing your urine or for testing your blood. Any blood glucose level above 15 mmol/l indicates that you should also check for ketones, but if your blood glucose level is usually very tightly controlled, you may find that ketones appear at lower levels, such as around 12 mmol/l.

A positive ketone test means that you are becoming acutely short of insulin and need to take action quickly. You should double your correction doses until the ketones disappear, and if in any doubt, seek medical help. Your diabetes team will help you identify when and how you can use ketone testing with your pump to ensure that you are able to manage your blood glucose levels.

Successful Diabetes Tip

Avoid ketoacidosis by ensuring your insulin supply is not interrupted for more than two hours at a time and by giving correction doses and increasing your basal rates during times when your blood glucose is too high

Chapter 6: Adjusting your insulin doses

One of the biggest influences on the difference pump therapy can make to your diabetes is based on your own adjustment of your insulin doses. This includes your basal rates, your food boluses and your correction doses. It also includes proactively adjusting insulin to prevent unwelcome situations such as hypoglycaemia occurring. This chapter looks at adjustments you can make, and how you can deal with situations that require more thought.

Adjusting your basal rate

If your basal rate is set correctly, your blood glucose levels before meals and before bed should stay within your target range. To assess individual parts of the day, take your blood glucose no more than three hours apart to identify if your insulin dose is correct. Also, look for patterns of higher or lower blood glucose readings at different times of the day. If you want to test how well your basal rate is working over a mealtime, eating a carbohydrate-free meal will mean that you don't need to give any boluses that could have an effect on your blood glucose levels.

Because the doses you are dealing with are small, for example you might be taking 0.8 units of insulin per hour, the adjustments should also be small ones, for example increasing or decreasing by 0.1 unit per hour, at least until you grow in confidence.

As a general rule, if your blood glucose is too high at a certain point in the day, you need to adjust your dose **the hour before** the high reading, and in some cases you may also need to alter the hour prior to that. Changing no more than three consecutive hours at a time, and waiting a day or two to see the effect, will help you avoid your blood glucose starting to swing high and low.

If you find you are getting low blood glucose levels at certain points in the day, and you are finding that lowering your basal rate is not being effective, it may mean that you have not lowered it early enough. You should also expect that your doses will dramatically vary between two consecutive hours. For example, if you were taking 0.8 units in one hour, then having 0.1 unit the next hour to avoid hypos, you will probably get a better effect by altering them to 0.5 units and 0.4 units per hour, giving you the same amount of insulin but reducing the dose slightly earlier.

Also, your pump will give you the option of programming more than one basal rate, which can then be stored in the memory or downloaded onto your computer. This gives you the flexibility of using different rates on different days – for example your insulin requirements on work days might be very different from when you have a day off, or if you work varying shift patterns you can develop a specific basal rate to suit each one, rather than having to re-programme your pump each time. If you use this system, and you make changes to one of your basal rates, it is important to consider whether you also need to make changes to any of those stored in the memory.

Your pump will also have a temporary basal rate function, which gives you the option of increasing or decreasing your basal rate by a percentage for a time length of your choice, such as a few hours, without making more permanent changes to your main settings. This option can work well if you are being physically active and need less insulin, or if you are unwell for a short period and need to increase your basal rate. Your health professional will offer you guidance on how to get the best out of using a temporary basal rate, and also by experimenting you will find the rates that will work best for you.

Successful Diabetes Tip

Testing your blood glucose at two to three hourly intervals and making small adjustments to your basal rate, then checking how well that has worked before making further changes, is how to optimise the overall stability of your blood glucose level

Adjusting your insulin to carbohydrate ratio

Testing your blood glucose levels before meals, and again two hours after your meals, will help you to assess whether your insulin to carbohydrate ratio is working well. If the ratio is correct, your blood glucose level should be within 2 mmol/l of your pre-meal reading. If you haven't achieved this, you need to take a number of steps to identify what to do:

1. Check whether you have assessed the carbohydrate content of your meal accurately.
2. Find out whether this is a one-off situation or if it is happening on most days.
3. If it is a one-off situation, is there anything specific that might have affected your blood glucose level other than food, eg a variation in your usual physical activity level?
4. If it is happening frequently, check if it is happening with all your meals or just some of them.

If your carbohydrate assessment is accurate, and it is happening most days, then it is likely to be your insulin to carbohydrate ratio that isn't working for you. You then need to identify if there is a variation at different times of day, as your insulin resistance can vary through the day. You may find that you need to use different ratios for each meal, for example you may use a different ratio at breakfast time than you do when you eat your evening meal.

Once you have made changes to your insulin to carbohydrate ratio, using your blood glucose tests to find out if your new ratio works for you will help you identify if it has worked or if you need to make further adjustments. Experimenting is the key to gathering more information to help you keep in control of your diabetes.

It is also important to remember that the ratio that works for you is likely to change over time, such as when your body shape, activity levels or daily routines change, so it's worth setting aside time regularly to check that your ratios are still right for you or to adjust them if you need to.

Using different types of boluses

As already highlighted in chapter 3, your pump offers you a range of different ways in which you can give bolus doses of insulin, which are described in Table 9.

Table 9: Types of boluses

Type of bolus	Alternative terms	Description
Standard	Normal	A bolus that is delivered within a few seconds.
Extended	Square wave	A bolus that is delivered at a constant rate over a period of time decided by you, eg 30 minutes.
Mixed	Multi-wave Multi-phase Combo	A combination of a standard and an extended bolus, part given immediately and part given over a longer time period.
Split	Dual wave Dual phase	A bolus that is split into two standard boluses, with the amount and the timing decided by you.

Standard boluses, as previously discussed, are the easiest and quickest to use, and can be calculated for you by your pump. However, there are many situations, particularly related to your food intake and absorption, where other boluses might give you extra benefits and the opportunity to more tightly control your blood glucose, although it may take you time to become confident with using them.

To use different boluses in situations where your food may be absorbed more slowly, the first thing to remember is that you still use your usual insulin to carbohydrate ratio. You then programme your pump to give you insulin at the time the food you are eating has the greatest effect on your blood glucose level.

The times when you are likely to need a different type of bolus are:

* When your meal contains more than 50 grams of carbohydrate
* When the food you are eating has a low glycaemic index
* When your meal is high in fat, ie more than 15 to 20 grams in total
* When your meal is high in protein, ie more than 20-30 grams in total

Which bolus should I choose?

As a general rule, using an extended bolus isn't likely to be right for any meal, because you will need some insulin to be available immediately as your food starts to be digested. There are exceptions to this, for example if you have a specific condition such as gastroparesis where you cannot predict how effectively your food will be absorbed, in which case an extended bolus will probably be your usual choice.

So to have some insulin available, you will need a mixed or a split bolus. A good starting point would be to take around 70% of your total bolus immediately, and the remaining 30% either slowly or after a short period of time. If you use a mixed bolus, extending the delivery of 30% over an hour or possibly two hours should work, but you need to experiment with different foods and different timings to find out what is right for you. If you decide to take a split bolus, a gap of 30 to 45 minutes between the two boluses should be sufficient, although again that might vary with different types and amounts of food.

The other option you have is to still use the standard bolus setting but to take two boluses, rather than using the split bolus setting on your pump. This may be quicker to programme, but you then have to rely on your memory to take the second bolus.

Successful Diabetes Tip

Choosing a bolus that matches the type of food you are eating, as well as one that you find easy to use, is the secret to success in keeping your blood glucose levels within your target range.

Managing your insulin doses day to day

Although it may be possible to set your basal rates and boluses to match your usual routine, that doesn't take account of the variation in your days, where your insulin needs will vary from their usual amounts.

It's a matter of opinion whether you should avoid situations that cause fluctuations in your blood glucose levels in the first few days, or whether you should continue with your usual routine, and adjust your pump regimen to this from the start. For example, if you regularly work out in the gym three times a week, should you avoid this for the first few days or should you try and adjust your insulin pump doses to meet the challenge? There is no 'right way' as it will depend very much on how confident and prepared you feel for life with a pump. However, it is important to try and avoid hypos in the first few weeks, because hypos and the potential high blood glucose levels afterwards can make it extremely difficult to assess the effectiveness of the pump insulin doses you have chosen to give. Hypos are discussed in more detail on pages 57 to 59.

As a general principle, using your previous experience of managing your diabetes before you started using your pump will give you a baseline to work from. You can then apply this knowledge, alongside the new ways that you can manage your diabetes using your pump, to make your everyday decisions. Adopting a question-and-answer approach can be helpful to work out the best course of action. Tables 10 and 11 on the following two pages give examples of different situations to show how this can work.

Table 10: Adjusting insulin for a social situation

Situation: You are going to a party where there will be buffet food and you will probably have a few bottles of lager.	
Questions	**Potential answers**
1. What factors will influence your blood glucose level?	I will be eating over a longer period of time than my usual evening meal, and it might be difficult to work out the carbohydrate content of the buffet, so I'll have less control over that. Also the lager will probably raise my blood glucose level at first, but the alcohol will then make it drop later in the evening.
2. How would you have managed this type of situation before you had a pump?	I would have eaten some of the buffet and then at some point given an injection to approximately match the amount of food I ate. I would also have given less of my night-time long-acting insulin to try and prevent hypos during the night.
3. Did this work?	No
4. If no at step three, what went wrong?	I would normally have quite a high blood glucose level before bed, but treating that would give me a hypo during the night. I would also usually wake up quite low the next morning.
5. Using the pump settings, how can you create a more successful method of dealing with the situation?	I can give small boluses to match my food as I eat it, and give a small amount of insulin to deal with the initial effect of the lager. And I can reduce my basal rate overnight to avoid hypos.
Evaluation	
6. After you have experimented – what have you learnt worked for you using your pump?	This worked quite well but I was still a bit high before bed. No hypos during the night though! And my morning blood glucose level was quite good.
7. What do you plan to do next time?	I think I will bolus a bit more for my food, but I will also reduce my basal rate a bit earlier and keep it low throughout the night to avoid hypos.

Table 11: Adjusting insulin for a workout in the gym

Situation: You are going for your usual one hour exercise class after work, 6-7pm, before you go home for your evening meal.	
Questions	**Potential answers**
1. What factors will influence your blood glucose level?	The extra activity will make my blood glucose level drop.
2. How would you have managed this before you had a pump?	By having a high-energy bar and glucose drink before I started, plus another glucose drink at the end. I would then have given less insulin for my evening meal, and then maybe reduced my night-time insulin depending on my blood glucose level before I went to bed.
3. Was this successful?	Yes for most days, I had occasional hypos during the night.
4. Using the pump settings, how can you recreate the successful method of dealing with the situation?	I will try reducing my basal rate an hour before I start and keep the reduced rate on for the evening. Depending on how well that works, I will alter my evening boluses and overnight basal rate if necessary. So maybe I won't need to have so much extra food and drink.
Evaluation	
5. After you have experimented – what have you learnt worked for you using your pump?	This worked quite well, a reduced bolus and overnight basal rate helped me to avoid hypos. I still had a glucose drink after the class though, as my blood glucose level was only 4.1 and I didn't want a hypo.
6. What do you plan to do next time?	I will try reducing my basal rate a larger amount before and during the exercise class, so that hopefully I won't need that glucose drink at the end.

Whilst these examples might not have exactly matched the common situations you find yourself in, they have shown how you can alter your insulin doses more precisely with your pump, and so avoid relying on eating or drinking extra carbohydrate all the time to avoid hypos. It is unlikely that a single experiment will give you the answers, and many pump users report that it takes them around six months before they feel really confident about managing the pump in most situations.

Successful Diabetes Tip

Careful planning for different situations where you might need to alter your pump settings, and assessing how well they have worked, will help you build up experience and be more able to deal with anything unexpected that happens in your life.

Chapter 7: Living with your pump

There are many times when your usual daily routine will vary, and being proactive in working out how you will manage those situations will mean less hard work on the day. Over time, as you get more experienced with using your pump, planning for these situations will become easier.

Becoming your own detective

Whether you want to gain the most you possibly can from your insulin pump, or simply want it to make life with diabetes easier for you, the most important message to remember is that **insulin pump therapy is in your hands**. You will have lots of helpful input from others, and the education and advice you receive from your health professionals and from other pump users will be invaluable, but only you are able to make the essential day to day decisions.

As you will probably already have learnt (or will learn very early in your experience of using a pump), there is no perfect solution to any situation that will be successful every time. However, there are principles that can be followed in most situations, and over time, by experimenting, you will learn which of these principles are particularly helpful to you in particular parts of your life. This section looks at those principles and how they can help you.

Planning ahead

The more you think about how you are going to deal with what is coming up in your life, the more likely you are to succeed and to keep your blood glucose levels within the limits you want to. Going to a party where you are unsure what food and drinks will be available; taking part in long meetings; planning a strenuous mountain climb; or meeting a group of friends for a long lunch break – thinking about the best strategies to use ahead of time is helpful. Because you have an insulin pump, you will be able to adjust your insulin doses more proactively, in particular increasing and decreasing your doses before problems occur, rather than having to rely on extra food intake.

Using your blood glucose test results

Blood glucose testing is simply a way of finding out information that will help you to manage your diabetes more easily. For any situation you find yourself in, checking what effect it has on your blood glucose level will give you information that you can use to measure the success of your insulin management and also to plan for how you will manage the situation the next time it happens. So you might need to test before the event occurs, during it, and afterwards for as long as it may have an effect, to get the information you need.

Experimenting

Whether you 'live on the edge' with your diabetes or prefer to play it safe, experimenting with your pump is an important part of working out what is best for you and your diabetes. That does not mean that you have to put yourself at risk, but you may need to move out of your comfort zone a little bit to try new ways of managing your diabetes. For example, you may be used to eating at certain times to prevent hypoglycaemia, whereas with your pump, setting your basal rate to keep your blood glucose stable should mean that you can eat at times to suit you rather than your diabetes.

If you want to find out what works, plan ahead (as already discussed!), decide what you are going to try – for example using a temporary reduction in your basal rate to avoid the time you usually have a hypo – and test your blood glucose to see the effect. If it has worked, you can use that information to reset your basal rate for those few hours, again using your blood glucose test results to check the effect.

Proactive insulin adjustment

Thinking ahead about how you can alter your insulin dose to prevent difficult situations from happening in the first place is the road to success with your insulin pump. It is particularly useful if you find that different situations cause you to have frequent hypos or regular high readings, as it means that you can start to be in control of the situation instead of having to deal with it when it happens. Even if you feel you have got your blood glucose levels reasonably balanced, revisiting your blood glucose test results every few months, and fine-tuning your insulin doses, will give you maximum benefit from your pump.

Expect the unexpected

It is hard to be prepared for unexpected situations, but you never know what's about to happen in your life. For example if you decide to take your pump off for 30 minutes and go to the corner shop, you might find that something happens that delays you and you have no way of giving yourself insulin. So thinking about the 'what if' situations can be useful so that you can be as prepared as possible. For example, what if:

* Your cannula becomes dislodged
* Something happens to stop your pump from working
* You suddenly need more insulin during the day than you had anticipated
* You become unwell and your blood glucose rises dramatically
* You are delayed in getting home from work

There are probably other 'what ifs' that might happen in your life, or situations you can recall where you were unprepared. Because your pump only delivers rapid-acting insulin, you do not have any long-acting insulin to work in an emergency. It is therefore important to ensure that you have enough supplies with you to deal with any situation, from a pump failure to an unexpected event. Also, ordering your supplies in good time so that you don't run out unexpectedly, will mean you are prepared for anything.

Removing your pump

Whilst insulin pumps are designed for use over 24 hours each day, you can remove your pump for short periods. For example, you might want to remove your pump when showering or bathing, particularly if your pump is not waterproof. You might also want to take it off when undertaking physical activity such as swimming, contact sports, and sexual activity. There are also times when you might have to disconnect the pump, for example if you are having an X-ray, scan or some other hospital procedure, although it is worth asking if you can keep the pump on as policies vary in some hospitals.

Your pump will probably disconnect without you having to remove the cannula, and this is the recommended way to remove your pump, as it means that you can quickly reconnect and give insulin when needed.

The maximum amount of time recommended to disconnect is two hours. In many of the cases outlined above, the amount of time you have without your pump is likely to be only 20 to 30 minutes – if this is the case, the missed insulin is unlikely to have a significant effect on your blood glucose level. Working out how much insulin you have missed from your basal rate in the time the pump has been disconnected will help you make a decision about whether you need to take any action. Checking your blood glucose before you disconnect, when you reconnect and two hours later will enable you to identify any rises in your blood glucose level or whether you need to take a correction bolus.

If your pump is off for an hour or more, you are likely to need to make some adjustment to your insulin dose. Blood glucose testing is recommended as in the previous paragraph, and it is more likely that you will need a correction bolus. Over time, as you become more experienced, you might be able to work out how much correction bolus is needed and give it earlier than the two-hour point, therefore preventing your blood glucose from rising significantly.

If you need to disconnect for longer periods, for example if your pump stops functioning (which is highly unlikely but may still happen), or you are undergoing a hospital procedure where you cannot wear your pump, you need to be able to revert back to injection therapy. Your health professional will help you to identify what additional equipment and types of insulin you need to keep in case this happens, and keeping a written or computerised record of your average insulin doses will also help you calculate what doses you should inject. You are unlikely to need to return immediately to your pre-pump insulin doses as your time using the pump will probably have increased your insulin sensitivity, so using your current pump doses will be a better guide to the amounts you may need. If you are unsure how to work out your insulin doses, your diabetes team will be able to help you.

Illness

As you will already know, when you are unwell, your blood glucose levels become more difficult to control. This is because the illness and its effect on your stress levels, hormones and glucose production mean that your usual strategies for controlling your blood glucose levels are unlikely to be effective. This section looks at how you can keep on top of your blood glucose levels with your insulin pump, giving you one less thing to worry about whilst you are feeling unwell.

The main aim of managing illness is to prevent ketoacidosis, which was discussed on page 60. To do this, you need to start to alter your insulin doses as soon as you become unwell. So at the first sign of any illness, such as a cough, cold, sore throat or stomach upset, checking your blood glucose level every two to three hours will enable you to identify any rising levels. Giving correction boluses for any readings outside your target range will help you avoid very high blood glucose levels.

If your blood glucose levels are very high, such as above 15 mmol/l, testing for ketones will tell you if your body is becoming very short of insulin, and you may need to give larger correction doses. See the next section on ketoacidosis for more information on testing for ketones and what to do if you find you have them.

If you find that you need to give correction doses every two to three hours, consider whether it is worth adding more insulin into your basal rate as well, to try and prevent your blood glucose from rising so high and reduce your need for correction doses.

A temporary basal rate can deal with the immediate situation, and from using this, you can see whether it is adequate to prevent your blood glucose levels rising too high. A suggested starting point is to increase your basal rate to 130%, and check your blood glucose levels every two hours. If this does not have any noticeable effect, increase to 160% after two hours. This may still not be enough, as the effect of your illness is difficult to identify, so consider further increases.

If your illness does not go away within around 12 hours, or if you need to increase your basal rate by more than double, you will need to programme more insulin into your basal rate. It is recommended that you use a new profile, so that you can alter this as you need to during your illness but you still have your original one to refer back to and to revert to when you recover.

It can be worrying to see how much extra insulin you need if you are unwell, and it can be helpful to keep in mind that any percentage increases to your basal rate aren't necessarily large amounts. For example, if you have an hourly basal rate of 0.5 units, even if you double that rate you are still only taking an additional 0.5 of a unit. This is why alterations to your actual basal rate are likely to be required. Also, you cannot predict how much additional insulin will be needed for any type of illness, so try not to be apprehensive if you see your insulin requirements double, treble or even quadruple during an acute illness.

If you are taking a lot more insulin than usual, you may find that you need to change your infusion site more frequently than usual. Also, if you are giving a lot of correction doses but the insulin seems to be having very little effect, it may also be worth resiting your infusion set to make sure your insulin is being absorbed as well as possible. If you have taken two correction doses via your pump but your blood glucose is continuing to rise, it is recommended that you take your next correction dose using an insulin pen or syringe, and use a new injection site, to ensure the insulin is absorbed well.

If, as part of your illness, you suffer from nausea, vomiting or diarrhoea, this indicates that you are having difficulty absorbing the food you eat. If this is the case, you will still need correction doses of insulin, but it is worth being slightly more cautious about the amounts you take, because it will be difficult for you to treat a hypo if it occurs. It is important to keep drinking fluids as you can tolerate them. If you are not able to eat or drink for more than 24 hours or you are vomiting uncontrollably, seek medical help as you may need to go to hospital to avoid dehydration and ketoacidosis.

When you start to recover from your illness, you will probably find that your blood glucose will drop relatively quickly, for example over a 12 or 24 hour period. You will therefore need to reduce your insulin doses quickly to match this. You can reduce this gradually, or if you find you are having hypos, it may be easier to go straight back to your pre-illness doses, although you may still need to give some correction doses during the time you are recovering from your illness.

Physical activity

You will already be aware that you activity level will have an effect on your blood glucose. Knowing what is happening to your glucose stores and the amount of glucose you have available in your bloodstream can help you plan ahead to minimise this effect.

Whenever you increase your activity, even by relatively small amounts, glycogen is released from your liver and converted into glucose to give you extra energy. As your muscles use up this glucose during your activity, your blood glucose starts to fall. If the activity is quite intense, or it is prolonged over an hour or more, your blood glucose will drop more, increasing your risk of a hypo. And at the end of any activity where your liver has released glycogen, those stores will need to be replaced, which may take up to 24 hours or even longer for activities such as marathon running.

So to cope with these changes, in most circumstances you are likely to need to make changes to your food intake and your insulin doses. The changes you need to make for any activity depends on a number of aspects. The type of activity is important, also how intense it is, how long you do it for, and what time of day you choose to be active.

Your fitness level also has an effect – if you are quite fit generally, you will use your glucose stores more efficiently and so will probably need to make less adjustments, but if you are relatively inactive most of the time, then additional activity will require more proactive management.

Prior to using a pump, you may have found it easier to simply adjust your food intake to provide extra energy and avoid hypos, but with a pump, you can make proactive insulin adjustments that can make activity much easier to manage and so much more enjoyable.

Before you start your activity

It is important that your blood glucose level is not too high before you start your activity, as you are unlikely to have enough insulin available in your body to deal with the glycogen that will be converted to glucose. A lack of insulin at this point will mean that you blood glucose can rise quite steeply during the activity, making it more difficult for you to carry on. So for any blood glucose level above 11 or 12 mmol/l, a correction dose should be given, and the activity shouldn't be started until your blood glucose has dropped to closer to your usual levels. If you are undertaking moderate or intense activity (see the next sections for details), these should not be attempted if your blood glucose is above 14 mmol/l.

Depending on the level of activity you are undertaking, your plan of action will vary. The following examples provide suggestions of what might work in different circumstances.

Light activity

Examples: Housework
30 minutes walking
Supermarket shopping

Ideas on how to adjust insulin and/or food intake:

* Programme a temporary basal rate of 70% one hour prior to your activity and return to your normal basal rate immediately after your activity.
* OR eat 10 grams of carbohydrate, programme a temporary basal rate of 70% immediately before your activity, and return to your normal basal rate immediately after your activity.

Moderate activity

Examples: A game of golf
30 minutes running
1 hour swimming
1 hour tennis

Ideas on how to adjust insulin and/or food intake:

* Programme a temporary basal rate of 70% one hour prior to your activity and discontinue this one hour after the end of your period of activity.
* Also reduce your food boluses by about a third during the activity and for one or two hours after.
* You may also need a temporary basal rate of 80 to 90% for a further couple of hours following the activity.

Intense activity

Examples: 1 hour cycling
2 hours tennis
2 hours swimming
2 hours football

Insulin adjustment options:

* Programme a temporary basal rate of 50% one hour prior to your activity and continue this for two hours after the end of your period of activity.
* Following the above period, programme a temporary basal rate of 70 to 80% for up to a further 12 hours, or overnight if your activity was towards the end of the day.
* Reduce your food boluses by 50% during your activity and for one to two hours afterwards.
* Omit boluses completely during your activity for any snacks of 20 grams of carbohydrate or less.

It is also important to note that intense activity can be less predictable and also can greatly vary in terms of duration and energy use, so the insulin dose recommendations above are a guide only and are highly likely to need some adjustment to suit your specific needs.

Removing your pump for activity

The other option you have is to remove the pump completely during your activity. Whilst this may be unnecessary for the lighter types of activity, it may become a necessity if undertaking contact sports such as rugby or judo, or if swimming when your pump is not waterproof. If you decide to remove your pump, do this immediately before the activity starts, and keep the pump off for a maximum time of two hours. If you are undertaking a team sport, taking a blood glucose test at half time, reconnecting to give a bolus if needed, and eating a snack, can help you to manage the situation. You may still find that you need a temporary basal rate for a time after you reconnect, particularly if the activity has been intense.

After you finish your activity

Because your glycogen stores are being replaced, your blood glucose level in the hours following your activity can drop. Finding out what happens with your own blood glucose level by testing frequently can help you form a plan. This is particularly useful of you regularly undertake similar activity, for example go to the gym or play football once a week or more, as you can build up a plan of what works for you on the basis of the knowledge you gain from your blood glucose readings.

It is also important to note that sexual activity will have an effect on your blood glucose levels, in a similar way to other types of physical activity. It may be more spontaneous and be difficult to plan ahead, so a temporary basal rate in advance may not be practical, although it may be possible to programme one at the time. You can choose to keep your pump on during the activity or to take it off. If it is removed, remembering to reconnect it afterwards is an important aspect. You may also find you need 10 to 20 grams of carbohydrate afterwards to avoid hypos.

Alcohol

Dealing with the effect of alcohol on your blood glucose levels can be tricky. This is because your liver stores glucose from the food you eat, in the form of glycogen, which is converted back to glucose 24 hours a day as you need it. But when your liver is processing alcohol, it is less able to produce glucose on demand.

Having less glucose available has two potential effects. One is that your blood glucose may be significantly lower than usual, increasing your chances of a hypo. The second is that any hypos you do have may be more severe or even potentially life-threatening, because your liver is unable to come to the rescue with extra glucose.

The other factor that can make hypos dangerous is that it may be difficult for people around you to tell the difference between the effect of alcohol and whether you are having a hypo, so they may not identify your need for help as easily as usual.

So the main aim of managing your blood glucose when you drink alcohol is to avoid hypos, which may mean keeping your blood glucose level a little higher than usual to be safe. For example, if the blood glucose range you usually aim for is 4-6 mmol/l, you might raise this target to 7-10 mmol/l.

Prior to using your pump, you may have found it difficult to manage the times when you drink alcohol, and may have needed to eat large amounts of carbohydrate to counteract its effects. But with a pump, you can make many more proactive alterations to your insulin doses to have the effect you want on your blood glucose level. The following information provides some ideas on how you can manage your insulin doses using your insulin pump when drinking alcohol.

Before you start drinking alcohol

In the few hours before you start to drink alcohol, you could take a reduced amount of insulin for any carbohydrate you eat. This means that you start with a higher blood glucose than your usual level. Reducing any meal bolus by around 20% an hour or two before you start drinking is a good starting point.

Taking insulin for any carbohydrate in alcohol

Secondly, thinking about the type of drink you choose will help you identify a strategy, as follows:

- Drinks containing carbohydrate, such as beer, lager, cider or alcopops: these may give you a slight rise in your blood glucose for the first couple of drinks. If you decide you want to avoid this rise, you can take boluses of insulin for each drink, but it is important to only do this for the first 2 units of alcohol, because after that the alcohol will start to affect how efficiently your liver can convert glycogen, so your blood glucose from that point is likely to start dropping. Alternatively, you can give no boluses for these drinks, as your blood glucose will start to drop a little while later.
- Drinks containing either no carbohydrate or a very small amount, such as wine and spirits: these won't cause a rise in your blood glucose level so you won't need any boluses of insulin.

Avoiding post-alcohol hypoglycaemia

Two units of alcohol are unlikely to cause hypoglycaemia later on, but if you are drinking more than this, taking action to avoid hypos during the night is recommended. A temporary reduced basal rate is the easiest way to achieve this, which you can start whilst you are drinking (or even beforehand) and maintain it overnight overnight. A good starting point is a reduction of your basal rate by 30%, and you can use your blood glucose readings to identify how well your strategy has worked and make a plan for the next time you drink alcohol.

Eating carbohydrate whilst you are drinking

If you are eating small amounts of carbohydrate during the time you are drinking, such as 15-20g carbohydrate in a packet of crisps, it may be worthwhile omitting your bolus completely. For larger amounts, for example if you are out for dinner or eating buffet food at a party, a good strategy is to reduce your bolus amounts by around 50% to avoid hypos. As with changes to the basal rate, your blood glucose readings will tell you how successful it has been.

Taking your activity level into account

The amount of activity you are undertaking will also need to be taken into account. Sitting in a pub talking with friends won't use a lot of energy, but dancing at a party will, and also any sexual activity will take energy. If you use more energy, to keep safe from hypos you will probably need to reduce your basal rate even more than already recommended – so instead of reducing by 30%, you may decide to reduce by 50%.

Dealing with the longer-lasting effects of alcohol

Finally, you may find that the alcohol has a continued effect on your blood glucose the next day, which can continue for up to 48 hours, particularly if you have had a lot of alcohol. So keeping a close watch on your blood glucose level, and reducing your basal rate if you find your blood glucose is lower than usual, should be enough to counteract this effect.

Experimenting with these strategies or others you have identified should, over time, give you insight into what works best for you to avoid hypoglycaemia without major blood glucose level swings. Table 12 summarises the main aspects to think about to keep your blood glucose well-balanced when you are drinking alcohol.

Table 12: Strategies to maintain your blood glucose balance when drinking alcohol

* Possibly reduce your insulin beforehand * Give minimal boluses for the first couple of drinks containing carbohydrate * Reduce your basal rate overnight * Give smaller boluses than usual when drinking * Reduce your basal rate more if you are dancing or using a lot of energy * Consider whether you need to reduce your basal rate the next day * Use your blood glucose readings to assess the effect and proactively adjust your insulin or carbohydrate intake

Holidays

Going on holiday and being away from home will be made much easier and more enjoyable if you think in advance what you need to do to manage any situations you might come across.

Before you go

Firstly, when you are getting ready to go on holiday, check your pump supplies to make sure you have enough, as well as your insulin and blood glucose testing equipment. Taking more than the amount you need is recommended, for example you may need to change your infusion site more frequently if you are swimming a lot.

It is also worth checking your back-up supplies of injectable insulin in case you need to stop using your pump for any reason whilst you are away, which may be a quicker solution than trying to sort out something that has gone wrong with your pump. Does your insulin pen still work? Do you have some longer-acting insulin within its expiry date? Do you have enough supplies of non-pump insulin to last you for your holiday if you need it?

Other useful things to take are the telephone numbers of your pump manufacturers, including, if you are travelling abroad, the number of the pump manufacturer in the country that you are travelling to. This means that you can easily contact them if you have any major problems whilst abroad, for example if you need a new pump. Not all pump manufacturers will have offices in every country in the world, so you may find you are travelling to a country where health professionals are unfamiliar with your pump.

Table 13 on the next page provides a checklist that you can use to make sure you have everything you need.

Table 13: Holiday supplies checklist

Spare pump batteries
All disposable pump supplies (eg cannulae, tubing, insertion devices, insulin reservoirs)
Pump manufacturers contact details (UK and abroad if required)
Medical certificate or letter
Insulin for your pump
Longer-acting insulin with injection devices (either syringes or insulin pen and needles)
Rapid-acting carbohydrate for the journey
Blood glucose testing equipment
Ketone testing equipment
A written record of the type of insulin you use, your usual basal rate and your current ratios for food boluses and correction boluses.
Basic information about your diabetes and your pump in the language of the country you are visiting.

Travelling abroad

If you are flying, check with your airline beforehand about what rules they have about what you are able to carry in your hand luggage. It is also useful to take a letter or medical certificate from your doctor or your diabetes team, explaining about your insulin pump and also what supplies you need to have available at all times. Your pump can be taken safely through the airport scanners, and many pumps now have a 'flightsafe' mode they can be switched to for the duration of the flight. Once you are onboard the aircraft, it is also worth alerting the cabin crew to your insulin pump, so that they know what your needs are and won't be alarmed if they see you using your pump.

Taking the name of your insulin written down is useful, and you can also check with your diabetes team or direct with the insulin manufacturer to find out what the insulin is called in the country that you are visiting.

If you are crossing time zones, it is a good idea to have a plan of how you will manage your basal rate during the journey, particularly when the time of the country you are visiting is more than two hours different from your own, and when your basal rate varies greatly from one hour to the next. For time differences of two hours or less, simply adjusting the time setting on your pump to the local time in the country you are visiting, either during or immediately after your journey, will be sufficient to avoid excessive swings in your blood glucose levels.

If the time zone difference is greater than two hours, if your basal rate is similar over the hours you may simply be able to change the time setting on your pump, but if you have a bigger variation, you may need to be more proactive, and work out what changes you want to make to give yourself enough insulin but avoid hypos. Lowering your basal rate slightly, perhaps by using a temporary basal rate, and giving correction boluses for any blood glucose levels out of your target range, is one method of managing the flight. Another option is for you to set a standard basal rate for the whole flight, again giving correction boluses if necessary – if you choose this option, using a different basal rate profile means that you still have your original settings saved.

During or at the end of your journey, adjusting the time setting on your pump to match the local time means that your basal rates will be the same as when you are at home for each hour of the day, although anecdotally not everyone does this. You are likely to have erratic blood glucose levels to some extent in the 24 hours following your journey, so if you are only staying for 24 to 48 hours, it may not be worth changing the time setting.

Whilst you're away

Carrying carbohydrate-rich snacks, both when you are travelling and during your holiday, is a way of making sure you always have something on hand to treat a hypo, particularly if you aren't fluent in the language of the country you are visiting. This will prevent you trying to treat a hypo with, for example, a sugar-free drink.

Your blood glucose testing results will be vital to help you work out if your diabetes is as well-controlled as you want it to be, and be able to make the day-to-day decisions about your insulin pump doses.

If you are travelling to a country with a hot climate, you will have an increased chance of having a hypo, so you may need to reduce your basal rate to compensate, and also you may find that you need smaller food and correction boluses than usual. The tubing of your insulin needs to be kept out of the sun, as it can heat up quickly and if your insulin is warm, it may not be as effective as it usually is.

You may need to think carefully about where you position your cannula, so that it is out of the sun whenever possible. If your pump is waterproof you will be able to keep it attached for swimming, but otherwise if you need to detach it, make sure it is kept safe at all times – even though it is no use to others, it may look like an attractive item that could be stolen. If you want to swim for longer periods of time, re-attaching your pump and giving a top-up bolus every couple of hours can replace your basal rate. The tape that holds your cannula in place should stay attached, but check this frequently to make sure it has not started to come off.

For a cold weather holiday, your pump should be kept close to your body to ensure your insulin doesn't freeze, so for a skiing holiday, for example, you would keep your pump inside your ski suit. The functioning of your blood glucose meter may also be affected by the cold weather. Checking with the manufacturers of your pump and your blood glucose meter will give you information about the lowest temperature in which they will operate reliably, which will help you decide how you can use them during your holiday.

It's also worth remembering that there are many different factors that will make your blood glucose rise or fall more than usual when you're on holiday. Eating different foods, being more or less active than you usually are on a daily basis, having lower (or in some cases higher!) stress levels, can all contribute to your blood glucose level being erratic. Planning ahead to identify what effect you anticipate the plans for your holiday will have on your blood glucose level and how you can adapt your insulin doses to match, testing frequently, and taking action on the results, will all help prevent your diabetes from getting in the way of you enjoying your holiday.

A holiday from your pump?

You may decide that you want a holiday from your pump whilst you are away. This has some advantages, such as being able to swim, sunbathe and wear more skimpy clothing without having to worry about what is happening with your pump. But there are also some downsides, such as your blood glucose levels being less predictable, leading to your holiday being less enjoyable because of the amount of time you have to spend looking after your diabetes.

If you do decide to have a holiday from your pump, you may need to work with your health professional, family or friends to work out what insulin doses to inject. It is also recommended that you still take your insulin pump on holiday, in case you have a lot of difficulty controlling your blood glucose levels when you're taking injections again. You may feel you might not want to check your blood glucose levels very often, but it is good to have plenty of supplies so that you can if you want to.

Even if you have decided not to have a holiday from your pump, it is useful to have a written record with you of the insulin doses you will take if you need to stop using your pump for any reason. This means that you can easily switch to injections if necessary without your holiday being interrupted too much.

Successful Diabetes Tip

Planning ahead what you need to take on holiday, and how you are going to manage your diabetes and your insulin pump doses whilst you are away, will help prevent your diabetes from taking over your holiday.

Frequently Asked Questions

This section answers specific questions that may be on your mind when you wonder about, start or live with an insulin pump. Some summarise information from different places in the book and others deal with more specific situations not covered elsewhere.

Can I have a shower with my pump on?

If your pump is waterproof you can shower with it on, but most pumps are classed as 'splashproof' rather than waterproof, so you would need to disconnect your pump before you shower, and to reconnect it again afterwards. You can leave your cannula in whilst you shower – no insulin will leak out – or you might choose this time of day to put a new cannula in (although you probably won't need to resite it every day). If you remove your pump and switch it to 'stop mode', it may beep at regular intervals to tell you it's not giving you insulin – your pump doesn't know it's not connected! – so you might need to warn others around to expect the beeps.

What would I do with my pump if I wanted to have sex?

Whilst it may not be the most romantic situation, you need to plan what you do with your pump during sexual activity. You might choose to disconnect for a while, and simply reconnect the pump a little later, or you might decide that you feel more secure with your pump still connected, and you and your partner can work out together how best you can manage that. Asking other people on pumps how they manage will also give you plenty of practical ideas.

I'm fed up with carrying a rucksack around with all my supplies in – what can I leave at home?

The bottom line is that only you can decide on this. The minimum you should have available would be supplies to deal with anything going wrong with your pump or your infusion site, which in practical terms would mean the following:

- A new cannula
- Tape (if you need more tape than is supplied with the cannula).
- An infusion set
- An insulin reservoir
- Insulin, including enough to prime a new infusion set if necessary
- Equipment to inject insulin if your pump fails, eg a syringe or an insulin pen with needles.

There are many other supplies that you could carry, or that you should be able to get hold of within an hour or two, such as spare batteries for your pump, which can fail quite quickly even though your pump will warn you that the batteries are low, and ketone testing equipment. You might also want to keep a conversion chart handy in case you need to revert back to injections at short notice.

It's important to remember that you don't necessarily have to carry all this around. You might, for example, keep duplicate supplies at work, in your car, or at the houses of frequently-visited friends or relatives. This can be a way of avoiding taking everything with you, although it's important to remember to replace anything you've used in an emergency.

I have gastroparesis, which means that I never know if my food is going to be absorbed or not – how should I manage my insulin doses?

The main strategy likely to work for you is to use extended boluses for all your food. That way, none of your bolus will be absorbed immediately, and if you find your food isn't being absorbed you can cancel the remainder of the bolus at any time. You would need to extend the bolus over a longer time than most people, such as a minimum of 30 minutes and potentially up to two hours.

The good news about using an insulin pump with gastroparesis is that if you manage to achieve better blood glucose control, this can improve your gastroparesis to some extent, although it is unlikely to disappear completely. If you find that you do see improvements and your food is being absorbed more readily, you could start to give a small amount of your bolus immediately, but you would still probably need to be cautious. A bolus of no more than 20% given immediately, and 80% still extended for a period of time, is recommended.

At times, I have to take steroids for a few weeks or more, which always makes my blood glucose difficult to manage – what should I do with my insulin pump doses?

For times like these, where your blood glucose might be significantly higher than usual, a temporary basal rate is unlikely to be enough to control your blood glucose level. However, it might be a useful starting point to find out how much extra insulin works for you. By increasing your basal rate and testing your blood glucose level every few hours, you will be able to see how much effect it has. Whilst you are experimenting, you will probably still need to give correction doses, but over time you may be able to identify the basal rate changes you need to prevent your high readings, rather than simply taking action when they occur.

Longer term, if you can identify your usual insulin requirements when you are taking steroids, you can programme these into a different basal rate profile, so that you can easily revert to this profile whenever you need to take steroids. This doesn't mean that it will perfectly match your insulin needs every time, but it will provide a starting point. It also means that you can save your original basal rate for when your steroids stop.

You will also need to pay attention to the boluses – you are likely to need a larger correction ratio and a larger insulin to carbohydrate ratio. The main message is not to be scared of making big changes in your insulin doses – as long as you are able to test your blood glucose frequently, and can act quickly to catch any hypos early, you will reap the rewards of not having long periods of high blood glucose readings.

I'm planning to get pregnant in the next year or two – will I still be able to use my pump when I'm pregnant?

Yes, many people actually convert to using an insulin pump during their pregnancy because it can be easier to get very tight control of your blood glucose levels without as many hypos. It is important to be confident about putting your insulin doses up quickly if your blood glucose levels rise, particularly towards the end of your pregnancy when you could need around three times your pre-pregnancy insulin doses. Your specialist team will be able to help you work out how to manage your pump during pregnancy, labour and immediately after the baby is born.

I'm going into hospital for an operation on my knee and will need a general anaesthetic – will I be able to continue using my pump?

Hospitals vary in their policies around insulin pumps, but in theory there is no reason why you shouldn't keep your pump on for the whole of your stay in hospital. If possible, talk to the relevant staff beforehand and find out what their usual policies are. You will obviously not be able to adjust your insulin doses whilst you are under general anaesthetic, so the anaesthetist will need to take responsibility for your pump, but it can be much easier to control your diabetes by keeping your pump on than it previously would have been using an intravenous infusion of glucose and insulin. Your diabetes team may need to get involved to help the ward staff and operating department staff understand more about insulin pump therapy.

My 6 year old daughter has terrible hypos, and our diabetes team have advised that she should try pump therapy – is that a good idea when she is so young?

Pumps can be used at any age, even in babies of under a year old, so she certainly isn't too young. Your daughter will probably adapt very quickly to life with a pump, and your diabetes team will help ensure that both you and her become confident in your respective roles in terms of her diabetes, as well as helping you to work out how she will manage at school and in other situations. She is also much less likely to experience severe hypoglycaemia if she uses a pump.

Are there any particular legal restrictions or recommendations in relation to driving?

The laws around which vehicles you can or cannot drive when you take insulin are the same whether you use an insulin pump or take injections. Testing your blood glucose level before you drive, stopping every couple of hours to re-test, and making sure you have plenty of hypo supplies are the main things to remember. Also, some pump users report that if their seat belt rests immediately over their infusion site it can be uncomfortable, which might be worth bearing in mind, particularly if you are going on a long journey.

I've been asking my diabetes team about getting a pump for a while now, and it looks like it'll be happening soon, but what if I get it and find I don't like it?

Changing to taking your insulin via an insulin pump is very similar to when you try out a different insulin regimen – it should be seen as an experiment rather than a definite solution. More planning and preparation is involved in you starting to use a pump than there is to simply changing the type of insulin you take, which can make you feel pressurised to make it work, but this pressure is an illusion rather than a reality. So if you are unhappy with wearing or managing your pump, or if it doesn't seem to be working for your diabetes in the way that you hoped it would, it is fine to revert back to injections.

I have a very varied routine at work, no two days are the same and it's very unpredictable, it's always difficult to control my diabetes with injections and I have to change my insulin doses a lot. Will it be as difficult when I have a pump?

It is true that you will still need to vary your insulin doses to suit your varied work routine, but there's every chance it will actually become easier with an insulin pump. Having different basal rate profiles set for the different situations you find yourself in is one option, so that you simply switch from your usual basal rate to a different one as you need it. Using a temporary basal rate increase or decrease is another way that you can meet your varying needs. It can take time to work out what is the best action to take, and the more unpredictable your routine, the longer that might take, but you should in the long-term be able to find a system that works for you without having to experience your blood glucose levels swinging or being too unpredictable.

In conclusion

This book has provided realistic information and lots of practical advice on how you can make the most of insulin pump therapy. It has hopefully given you a detailed picture of the opportunities and ways of experimenting with insulin pump therapy to help you get the most out of it. Your own diabetes team will also provide help, information and advice, and there are many other websites, books and sources of information out there, many of which have been referred to in the book.

I hope all this information combined helps you realise your goals and aspirations in relation to pump therapy and your diabetes, and wish you the very best of luck for the future.

Thank you for purchasing this book, we hope you have enjoyed it and found it useful.

Please visit our website www.successfuldiabetes.com to see our ever expanding range of information and products.

The Successful Diabetes Team.

Printed in Great Britain
by Amazon.co.uk, Ltd.,
Marston Gate.